Interstitial Lung Disease

C. A. C. Pickering, MB, MRCP, DIH, MFOM
Consultant Thoracic Physician, Wythenshawe and
Withington Hospitals, Manchester

L. Doyle, MB, B.CH, FRCPI, DCH
Consultant Thoracic Physician, Wythenshawe and
Manchester Chest Clinic

K. B. Carroll, MB, CH.B, MRCP
Consultant Thoracic Physician, Wythenshawe Hospital
and Manchester Chest Clinic

Published,
in association with
UPDATE PUBLICATIONS LTD., by

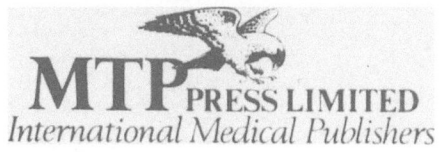

MTP **PRESS LIMITED**
International Medical Publishers

Published,
in association with
Update Publications Ltd., by

MTP Press Limited
Falcon House
Lancaster, England

Copyright © 1981 MTP Press Limited
Softcover reprint of the hardcover 1st edition 1981

First published 1981

ISBN-13: 978-94-009-8086-0   e-ISBN-13: 978-94-009-8084-6
DOI: 10.1007/978-94-009-8084-6

Contents

1. The Pneumoconioses

Pneumoconiosis is a generic term applied to a group of diseases caused by the inhalation of inorganic (mineral) dusts. These dusts are classified into two groups according to the pulmonary response: the non-fibrogenic (benign) and the fibrogenic pneumoconioses.

Non-fibrogenic (Benign) Pneumoconioses

The dusts of this group, providing they are free of toxic impurities, do not cause significant formation of reticulin fibres or give rise to collagenous fibrosis.

Types of Benign Pneumoconioses

The various mineral dusts causing benign pneumoconioses include:

1. Iron (siderosis)
2. Tin (stannosis)
3. Barium (baritosis)
4. Antimony
5. Cerium (rare earth element)
6. Chromite.

Clinical features. There are no specific symptoms or physical signs due to the inhalation of these dusts.

Lung function. No abnormalities of lung physiology are attributable to the inhalation of these dusts.

Radiology. Characteristically opacities from 0.5 to 4.0 mm in diameter are distributed through the lung fields. The density of these opacities varies with the atomic number of the mineral, barium, with an atomic number of 56, forming extremely dense opacities.

Prognosis. This group of pneumoconioses produces radiographic abnormalities which are not associated with symptoms, clinical signs or impairment of lung function and do not affect the life expectancy of the individual.

Fibrogenic Pneumoconioses

Asbestos-induced Lung Disease

The fire resistant properties of asbestos have been known since early times (Plutarch AD 510, Pliny AD 70), but its commercial development did not commence until 1880. By 1940 production of asbestos fibre had become large scale (500,000 tons per year) and in 1970 this had increased to three million tons per year. The major sources of asbestos are the Quebec province of Canada, the Ural mountains in the USSR and Southern Africa.

Asbestosis was first recognized in 1907 (Murray), but it was not until 1930, following the report of Merewether and Rice, that safety measures were adopted by factories and the medical surveillance of workers developed. The carcinogenic behaviour of this mineral fibre has only been fully appreciated over the last 20 years.

Physical Characteristics of Asbestos

Asbestos is a generic term applied to some of the fibrous mineral silicates. It is their varying chemical composition and physical structure which determines both their industrial uses and their ability to cause lung disease. Asbestos comprises two groups of minerals (Table 1).

The most important commercial fibres are chrysotile (90 per cent of world asbestos production), crocidolite and amosite. The

Table 1. The asbestos groups of minerals.

Serpentine group	Amphibole group
Chrysotile (white asbestos)	Crocidolite (blue asbestos)
	Amosite
	Anthophyllite
	Actinolite
	Tremolite

fibres of chrysotile are long, soft, and tend to curl; this physical structure leads to greater deposition higher up the bronchial tree. In contrast to chrysotile, the fibres of crocidolite are short and straight and are able to penetrate deeper into the acini of the lung, beyond the reach of mucociliary clearance.

Uses and Exposure to Asbestos

Asbestos has a wide variety of uses in industry. Of particular importance are asbestos cement products (roofing material, pipes and sheets), floor tiling materials and its use for heat insulation and fireproofing.

Exposure to asbestos fibre may occur as a result of:

1. Industrial exposure. In previous years the greatest exposure occurred in the crushing, bagging and spinning of asbestos. With modern factory safety standards exposure in the asbestos industry itself is lower.

2. Para-industrial exposure. Workers in this group are exposed to significant levels of asbestos and only careful history taking will reveal their past exposure. The workers may not have used asbestos itself, but worked as maintenance fitters, joiners, welders or electricians in areas where asbestos fibre is used. The removal of old asbestos insulation by 'strippers and laggers' may result in heavy exposure to fibre in workers who are not usually adequately protected.

3. Non-industrial exposure. Neighbourhood exposure has occurred in the past in the vicinity of asbestos mines and mills. Newhouse and Thompson (1965) identified the hazard to

housewives when laundering dust-contaminated clothing. In Finland residents in an asbestos mining area have a high incidence of pleural plaques and/or calcification.

Asbestos fibre once incorporated into manufactured products is relatively well bound and is unlikely to be a health hazard, providing the articles remain intact.

Clinical Features of Asbestos-induced Diseases

The following abnormalities may arise from asbestos exposure:

1. Diffuse interstitial pulmonary fibrosis (asbestosis).
2. Malignant mesothelioma of the pleura and peritoneum.
3. Pleural fibrosis and plaque formation.
4. Pleural effusion (benign).
5. Bronchial carcinoma.

Diffuse Interstitial Pulmonary Fibrosis (Asbestosis)

Definition

The term asbestosis was first suggested by Cooke (1924), when describing a case of pulmonary fibrosis associated with asbestos exposure. Here the term asbestosis refers only to fibrosis of the lung, and is not used in a generic sense to describe all asbestos-induced disorders.

Epidemiology

The incidence and prevalence of asbestosis in the UK is not accurately known. The numbers of new cases diagnosed for compensation are shown in Table 2. The increasing incidence of asbestosis probably reflects both a greater awareness of the disease and the heavy exposures which occurred in the industry 10 to 15 years ago. There is, however, no doubt that these figures underestimate the true position in the UK.

Table 2. Numbers of newly diagnosed cases of pneumoconiosis diagnosed in the UK by the Pneumoconiosis Medical Panels.

	1968–1972	1973	1974	1975	1976
Pneumoconiosis					
Coalmining	3,420	515	539	683	575
Other mining and quarrying	258	31	24	41	76
Pottery	140	16	15	24	17
Asbestos[1]	687	143	139	161	189
Diffuse mesothelioma: all cases[2]	442	104	142	148	191
Accompanied by asbestos	118	30	50	42	47
Beryllium poisoning	—	—	—	2	1

[1] Excludes cases where diffuse mesothelioma was also diagnosed.
[2] Includes pleural and peritoneal cases.
From DHSS, *Social Security Statistics,* HMSO, London, 1976.

Pathology

The distribution of the fibrosis is predominantly in the lower zones of the lungs. Macroscopically, in early disease patchy grey coloured fibrosis is seen. As the disease becomes more advanced these fibrotic changes become diffuse throughout both lower lung zones. Honeycombing may be present, and occasionally bronchiectasis is seen in areas of severe fibrosis. Rarely, large fibrotic masses are present usually in the lower zones.

Microscopically, lesions first occur in the alveoli of the respiratory bronchioles. Deposition of reticulum occurs around collections of asbestos fibre and macrophages. The reticulum fibres are replaced by collagenous fibrosis, leading to the obliteration of alveoli. Fibrosis gradually spreads peripherally to involve distal alveoli, leading to a widespread network of fibrosis. Asbestos bodies are seen in relation to the fibrosis. These structures are rod-shaped with clubbed ends, yellow-brown in colour and range in length from 10 to 50 μm and in width from 2 to 6 μm. Asbestos bodies consist of an asbestos fibre coated with a protein-like material and ferritin granules. The body results from the phagocytosis of the fibre by lung macrophages. Asbestos bodies are found in a high proportion of normal lungs at autopsy and are only indicative of exposure to asbestos fibre.

Pathogenesis

A number of theories have been proposed to explain the fibrogenic effect of asbestos fibre:

1. Direct mechanical irritation by the sharp asbestos fibre.

2. Solubility theory, fibrosis resulting from the direct leaching out of metal ions and/or silicic acid from the asbestos fibres.

3. Autoimmune theories. Abnormal globulins are either produced or localized by macrophages in the lung, resulting in an antigen–antibody reaction. The prevalence of circulating antinuclear and rheumatoid factors is high in asbestosis, 20 to 25 per cent of individuals with asbestosis having circulating antinuclear factor (ANF) and rheumatoid factor (Turner-Warwick and Haslam 1971).

None of these theories adequately explains the pathogenesis of asbestos-induced fibrosis. The initiation of fibrosis appears to depend on the disruption of the macrophage following phagocytosis of the asbestos fibre. It seems likely that the macrophage, either directly or as a result of releasing factors as yet unidentified, stimulates the fibroblasts, thus initiating fibrinogenesis.

Clinical Findings

Symptoms and signs are insidious in onset. Breathlessness on exertion, sometimes associated with a paroxysmal dry cough is a presenting symptom in most individuals. In the majority of patients the disease progresses, after cessation of exposure, leading ultimately to the development of cor pulmonale and death. There is now evidence that early detection and removal from contact with asbestos may arrest the progress of the disease. The time interval between exposure to asbestos and the development of symptoms is between 10 and 15 years, although with heavy exposure fibrosis may occur more rapidly.

The earliest physical sign of asbestosis is the presence of fine and persistent late inspiratory crackles, present in the dependent parts of the lungs. As the disease progresses these crackles become more widespread and are present throughout inspiration. Other adventitious sounds, such as wheezes, are unusual. Loss of weight is not a feature of asbestosis, except in advanced disease or when the disease is complicated by the development of a malignant mesothelioma or bronchial carcinoma.

Pulmonary Function Tests

The characteristic functional abnormalities are the progressive reduction of total lung capacity and vital capacity and impairment of gas transfer. The measurement of gas transfer and vital capacity are probably the most sensitive parameters for detecting early disease.

Airways obstruction is said to be uncommon, and when present is usually related to cigarette smoking and coexisting chronic obstructive airways disease. However, Fournier-Massey and Becklake (1975) reviewed 375 published cases of asbestosis and found airways obstruction to be a feature in a significant number of patients (29 per cent had features of either obstruction or mixed obstruction and restriction). Muldoon and Turner-Warwick (1972) have suggested that this airways obstruction may be due to involvement of the smaller airways in the fibrotic process.

Radiology

The first changes of asbestosis occur in the lower halves of the lung fields in the majority of patients, and in a significant proportion of cases they are associated with pleural changes (Figure 1). Fletcher and Edge (1970) describe the earliest changes as being accentuation of the small vessel markings associated with small linear opacities. These changes are best seen initially near the costophrenic angles. As the disease progresses, the fine linear opacities become thicker and more profuse. Finally, a honeycomb appearance develops in the lower zones with reduction of the area of both lung fields.

Nodular opacities may also be present but usually to a lesser degree. Rarely, large opacities occur, similar to those seen in complicated coal workers' pneumoconiosis. They are most commonly located in the lower zones. As in other types of diffuse

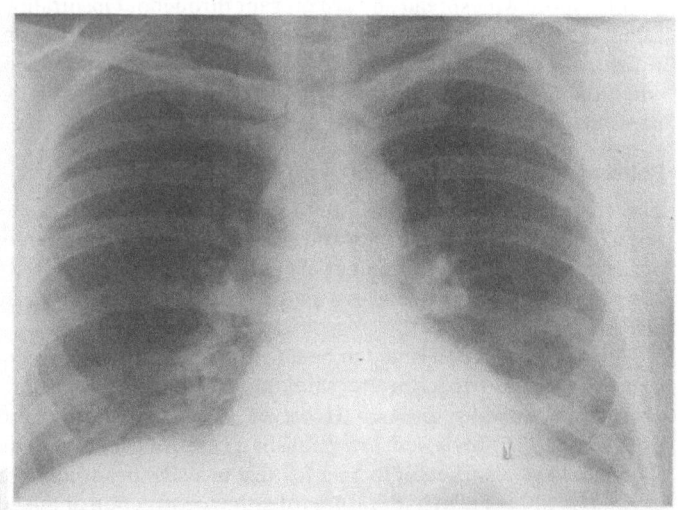

(a)
1967

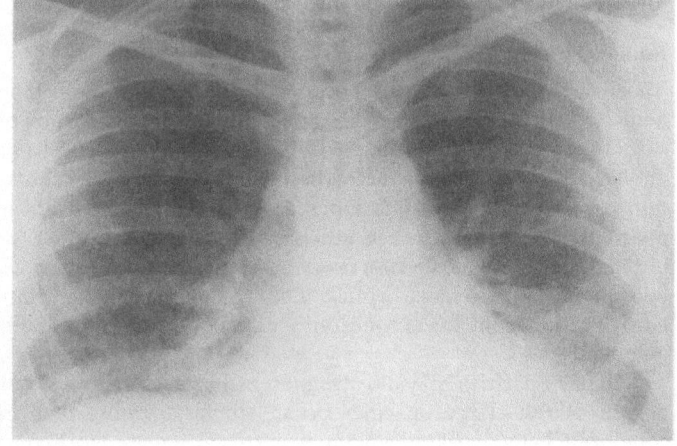

(b)
1971

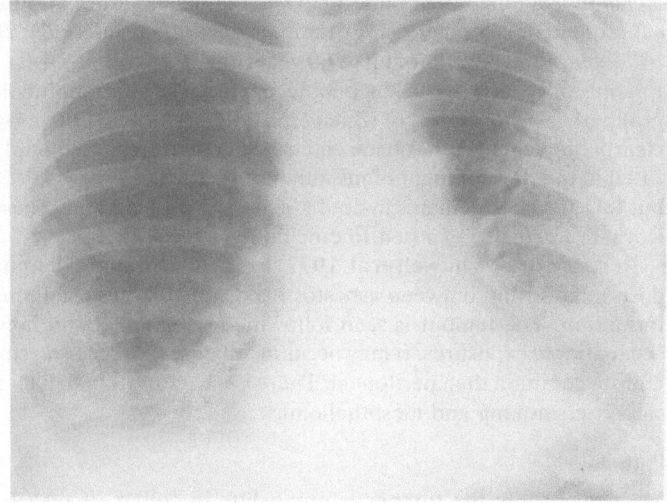

(c)
1974

Figure 1. *Radiographs showing progression of asbestosis over a 7-year period. The man had been employed as an asbestos weaver for 17 years. ILO category p type lesions are present in the lower zones in the 1967 radiograph. These rapidly increased in number and extended into the middle zones in the subsequent radiograph, the changes being most marked on the left. (Pleural plaques are present in the right midzone and some contraction of the left lung has occurred.)*

interstitial fibrosis, asbestosis may occur in the presence of a normal chest radiograph.

Malignant Mesothelioma of the Pleura

Introduction

An association between asbestos exposure and malignant mesothelioma of the pleura was first noted in 1946 by Wyers, but it was not until the report by Wagner and his colleagues in 1960, describing 33 cases of mesotheliomas in individuals who had had industrial and non-industrial exposure to the dust of crocidolite asbestos, that it became apparent that this was more than a rare association.

There is a long latent period between initial exposure and the subsequent development of the tumour; the average interval is 20 to 25 years and periods of up to 60 years have been reported. The tumour probably occurs in people exposed to the amphibole group of asbestos fibres, of which crocidolite asbestos is the most clearly implicated. It has been claimed that amosite is also implicated in the development of mesotheliomas (Selikoff et al. 1972) but this assertion remains in doubt, since it is probable that these workers were also exposed to crocidolite.

Recent work (Whitwell et al. 1977) has demonstrated a definite dose relationship between asbestos exposure and mesothelioma formation. The tumour is seen following occupational and non-occupational exposures. It may occur in either sex; the pleural site is more common than peritoneal. There is no association between cigarette smoking and mesotheliomas.

Pathology

Macroscopically the tumour is grey/white in colour; it may be localized to part of the surface of the lung or may encase the whole surface of one lung. The tumour has a tendency to spread along interlobar tissues. Microscopically, it is characterized by a variety of appearances, a number of which may be seen within a single tumour. Whitwell and Rawcliffe (1971) classified the tumour into four types: tubulopapillary, sarcomatous, undifferentiated polygonal and mixed. The commonest type is tubulopapillary, and considerable difficulties may arise in trying to distinguish this from secondary adenocarcinomas when a primary tumour has not been identified. The tumour may metastasize to lymph nodes and less commonly to other organs.

Pathogenesis

The pathogenesis of malignant mesothelioma in man is poorly understood. Animal experiments indicate that any type of asbestos fibre, as well as glass fibre, is capable of producing mesothelioma when inoculated intrapleurally. The finding in South Africa that the incidence of mesotheliomas varied widely between two areas in which crocidolite was mined, the crocidolite in the two areas being of the same chemical composition but of different physical characteristics, suggests that the physical characteristics of the fibre, and consequently its ability to reach the peripheral parts of the lung, may be the most important factor in determining the development of this tumour.

Clinical Findings

In the majority of patients developing pleural mesotheliomas, the onset of symptoms is insidious. Chest pain and breathlessness are the most common symptoms. The pain is dull and persistent and often interferes with sleep. Physical signs depend on the stage at which the patient presents. The patients are usually in good general health, finger clubbing is relatively rare (10 to 15 per cent of patients), and physical signs, if present, are those of a pleural effusion.

Diagnosis is made by needle or open lung biopsy.

Radiology

Pleural mesotheliomas present either as pleural effusions, or as irregular lobulated opacities on one chest wall, or as a combination of both. Involvement of the chest wall usually occurs without evidence of rib erosion, a distinguishing feature from adenocarcinomata which invade bone more frequently.

Diagnosis and Treatment

The diagnosis can only be made by tissue examination and, even when adequate biopsy material is available, this may be difficult. Often the definitive diagnosis is only made at postmortem examination. The presence of hyaluronic acid in pleural fluid provides some additional evidence in favour of malignant mesothelioma, although it may also be found in association with other malignant tumours of the pleura.

There is no curative treatment for this tumour and the outcome is inevitably fatal. The survival time, which is not significantly altered by radiotherapy, chemotherapy or surgical excision, is on average 15 months from the time of diagnosis.

Pleural Fibrosis and Plaque Formation

Two types of pleural reaction are associated with asbestos exposure: a diffuse pleural fibrosis involving both the parietal and
visceral pleura, and localized hyaline pleural plaque formation.

Pleural plaques and pleural fibrosis rarely give rise to respiratory symptoms. However, extensive pleural fibrosis is associated with abnormal lung function studies, chiefly a reduction in
lung volumes. Pleural plaques are found in the parietal pleura,
they are bilateral and occur more commonly in the lower zones of
the pleura and across the diaphragms. Plaque formation is associated with exposure to all types of asbestos fibre with an interval of
many years between exposure and radiographic evidence of
plaque formation. The prevalence of plaque formation is chiefly
determined by the duration rather than the intensity of asbestos
exposure. Their description in communities without occupational
asbestos exposures appears to be due to the presence of asbestos,
primarily tremolite, in the soil.

Histologically, plaques consist of collagenous connective tissue,
which is avascular, acellular and arranged as bundles of fibres.

Radiologically, plaques are best visualized on anterior oblique
views taken at 45°, and are more easily seen when they are
calcified. Calcification in the pleura may also arise following infection (tuberculous pleurisy), trauma and haemopneumothorax; in
these instances calcification is usually unilateral.

Pleural Effusion (Benign)

Pleural effusions may sometimes occur in asbestos workers,
usually presenting with pleuritic chest pain. The effusion may be
unilateral or bilateral, resolving spontaneously and often leaving
residual pleural thickening. It is a diagnosis of exclusion, the most
important diagnosis to be excluded being a malignant
mesothelioma.

Bronchial Carcinoma

The association between lung cancer and asbestosis has been
recognized since the 1930s. The incidence of lung cancer is

increased in both workers exposed to asbestos and in those who have developed asbestosis. It is not associated with any particular type of fibre. Autopsy studies of cases of asbestosis suggest that 15 to 20 per cent of these workers die from lung cancer. In Selikoff's series (1968) of insulation workers, he calculated that there was 92 times the risk of developing bronchial carcinoma in smoking insulation workers than in non-smoking, non-asbestos exposed workers. It is of interest that none of the 87 non-smoking asbestos workers in this series developed bronchial carcinoma. This study indicates that a major determinative factor in the production of lung cancer among asbestos workers is their cigarette smoking habits, carcinoma of the lung occurring only very rarely in non-smoking asbestos workers. Whitwell and co-workers (1974) have produced evidence that the distribution of tumour cell type is different from that seen in smokers not exposed to asbestos, with a predominance of adenocarcinomata.

Coal Workers' Pneumoconiosis (CWP)

Introduction

Coal workers' pneumoconiosis (CWP) results from the inhalation of coal dust. An identical disease is seen amongst workers exposed to graphite and to synthetic carbons. This pneumoconiosis is categorized into two forms, simple and complicated, according to the radiological appearance. Simple pneumoconiosis is present when opacities not exceeding 1 cm in diameter are present. If opacities greater than 1 cm in diameter are present, the disease is said to be complicated pneumoconiosis. The term progressive massive fibrosis (PMF) is synonymous with complicated pneumoconiosis.

Epidemiology

The prevalence of coal workers' pneumoconiosis has fallen significantly over the last 20 years with the advent of dust control measures. In the UK the prevalence of all categories of pneumoconiosis was 15.2 per cent in 1959, and 9.7 per cent in

1970. The development of progressive massive fibrosis is influenced by the radiographic category of pneumoconiosis present. Its incidence is increased in those with category 2 or more pneumoconiosis and by the geographical region in which the coalmine is situated. Certain types of coal, particularly anthracite, are associated with higher dust levels, and a higher prevalence of simple and complicated pneumoconiosis. McLintock and co-workers (1971) showed an expected attack rate of progressive massive fibrosis (PMF) of 1.5 per cent in active British miners with category 2 or more pneumoconiosis (see page 16).

Pathology

The characteristic lesion of CWP is the dust macule, which is distributed throughout both lung fields, predominantly in the upper lobes. The macule consists of dust and dust-containing macrophages, with small amounts of collagen and reticulin fibres. The dust particles concentrate around respiratory bronchioles, which themselves may contain large numbers of dust-containing macrophages.

Emphysema of centrilobular type may be seen in some coal macules.

The black fibrotic masses of progressive massive fibrosis (defined as a nodule greater than 1 cm in diameter) are found mainly in the posterior segment of the upper lobes or in the superior segment of the lower lobes. They are frequently bilateral and are variable in shape and size. The dust macules of simple pneumoconiosis are usually present, although on occasions they may be virtually absent.

The massive lesions consist of large amounts of dust and dust-laden macrophages and dense bundles of collagen and reticulum fibres. Bronchioles and blood vessels in the affected areas are obliterated.

Pathogenesis

It was believed for many years that the quartz content of coal dust was the major factor determining the category of simple pneumoconiosis and the development of PMF lesions. This hypothesis is not supported either by cases of simple pneumoconiosis and PMF occurring in workers exposed to carbon black, which contains minute amounts of quartz, or by the absence of any correlation between the quartz content of the coal dust and the prevalence of simple pneumoconiosis and PMF. The critical factor appears to be the total dust content of the lungs, but the mechanism which triggers the development of simple or complicated pneumoconiosis is not known.

Clinical Findings

Over the past 10 years there has been considerable controversy over the clinical significance of simple pneumoconiosis. On the basis of current evidence it may be said that simple pneumoconiosis neither shortens life nor causes disability. It is not accompanied by any specific symptoms. If symptoms of cough, sputum, wheeze or breathlessness are present, these are usually related to the cigarette smoking habits of the individual representing coincidental chronic secretory or obstructive bronchitis.

Progressive massive fibrosis, however, may be associated with both disability and a reduced life expectancy, particularly when it is category B or C (see page 18).

Pulmonary Function Tests

Minor abnormalities of pulmonary function in simple pneumoconiosis have been described: elevation of residual volume, ventilation–perfusion abnormalities, reduced diffusing capacity in the presence of p type opacities (see page 18) and abnormalities of frequency dependent compliance. These physiological abnormalities are very small, and are unlikely by themselves to be associated with respiratory symptoms or impairment of exercise tolerance. PMF, however, does result in impairment of ventilatory capacity and in airways obstruction in some, but not all, individuals.

Radiology (Figure 2)

Coalworkers' pneumoconiosis is categorized radiologically according to the ILO/UC Classification of Pneumoconiosis

(1971). Radiological opacities are classified first by size into small (up to 1 cm in diameter) and large opacities (1 cm or larger in diameter). Small opacities are further classified into categories 1, 2 and 3 according to the profusion of opacities in the lung fields. In category 1 radiographs opacities are present, but few in number; in category 2 radiographs numerous opacities are present with normal lung markings; in category 3 radiographs the opacities are very numerous with partial or complete obscuring of the lung markings. The opacities are then subdivided into groups by their shape, being either rounded or irregular. The rounded opacities

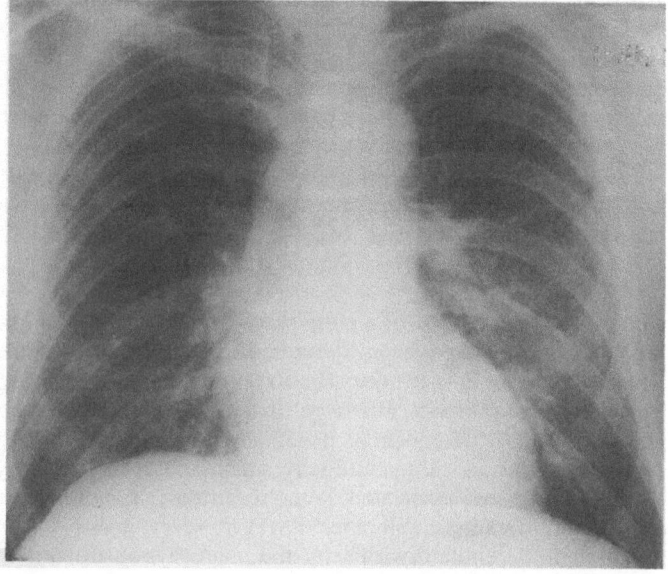

(a)

Figure 2. *Radiographs showing progressive coal pneumoconiosis in a miner who worked 41 years at the coal face. (a) The film in 1973 is ILO category 1p. (b) By 1979 early confluence is present in the right upper zone. Eggshell calcification of the hilar lymph nodes is also seen, (c) Tomography demonstrates an area of calcification in the PMF, a sign helpful in distinguishing this lesion from a bronchial carcinoma.*

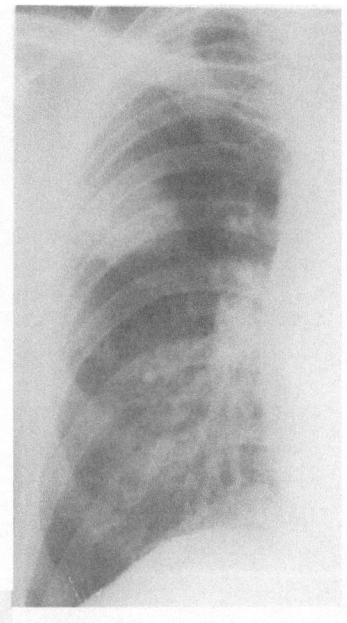

(b)

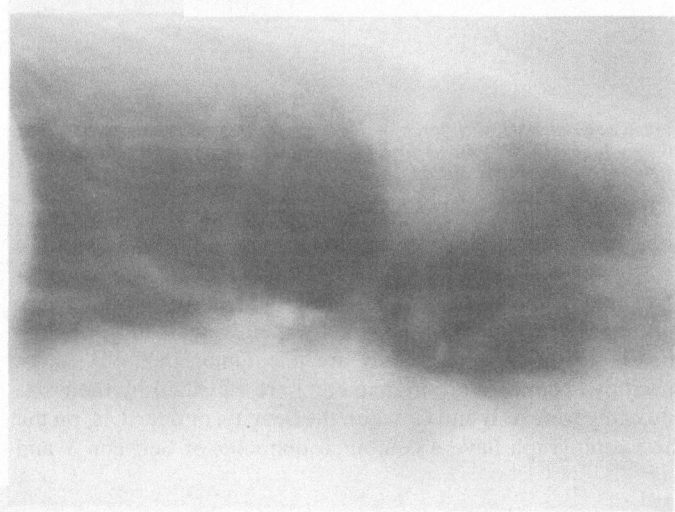

(c)

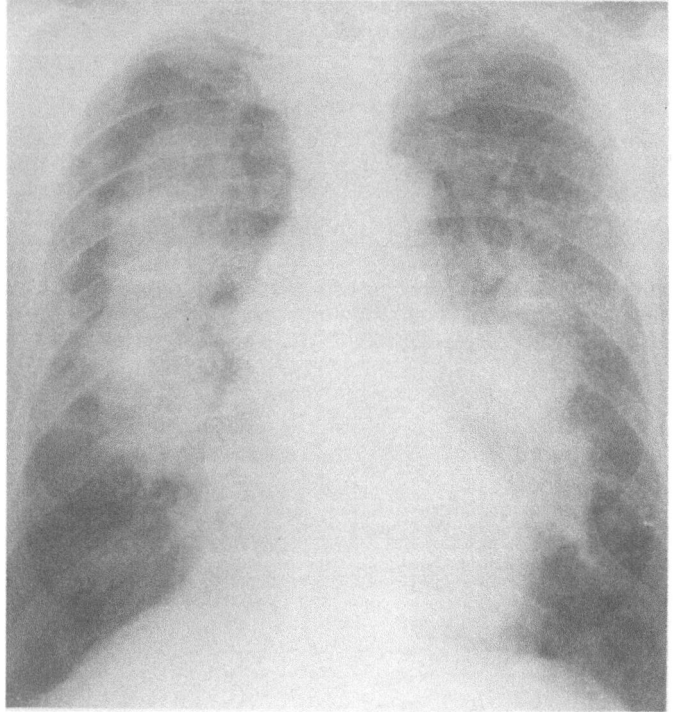

Figure 3. *Coal PMF with large, well circumscribed bilateral opacities in a miner who spent 47 years at the coal face. (By courtesy of the Manchester Pneumoconiosis Medical Panel.)*

are further separated according to size into p (up to 1.5 mm), q (1.5 to 3.0 mm) and r (3.0 to 10.0 mm) (Figure 3). Irregular opacities are divided into s (fine), t (medium) and u (coarse) types. Although irregular opacities are frequently seen in interstitial fibrosis due to asbestosis, they are uncommon in CWP. Large opacities (1 cm or more in diameter) are classified by their size into categories A, B and C. When the opacity, or opacities, on the chest radiograph have a combined diameter of between 1 and

5 cm, it is category A. Opacities whose diameters are greater than 5 cm, but less than one third of the lung field, are category B and those whose combined diameters exceed one third of the lung field are category C.

As a result of considerable observer variation in interpreting chest radiographs in CWP, the ILO issue a series of classified standard films. The films being read are then compared with these standard films. This classification can be used to classify all types of pneumoconiosis, including asbestosis.

The radiographic appearances of CWP correlate well with the coal dust content of the lungs. The earliest changes are of small, ill-defined opacities present in the upper and middle zones. When a category 3 stage is reached, the opacities are distributed throughout both lung fields.

PMF opacities may be unilateral or bilateral and tend to be localized to the upper and middle zones. They usually occur on a background of category 2 or 3 simple pneumoconiosis, although occasionally there is no evidence of simple pneumoconiosis.

Rheumatoid Pneumoconiosis (Caplan's Syndrome)

In 1953 Caplan described specific chest radiograph abnormalities seen in coal miners suffering from rheumatoid arthritis. There are no specific pulmonary symptoms associated with this syndrome. The characteristic radiographic changes are of multiple (occasionally single), rounded and peripherally situated opacities, varying in diameter from 0.5 cm to 5.0 cm, developing rapidly on a background of category 0 to 1 pneumoconiosis. Central necrosis followed by cavitation of the nodules is fairly common. The pathology of Caplan nodules is distinct from the pathology of both the nodules of CWP and silicosis. The nodules show concentric layers of dust, with central necrosis surrounded by an area infiltrated with lymphocytes and plasma cells. Calcification in the nodule is frequent.

The pathogenesis of these lesions is not clear but immunological factors may be involved. The sera of miners with rheumatoid pneumoconiosis with or without arthritis and in miners with PMF have increased levels of circulating rheumatoid factors and anti-nuclear factors. Since Caplan's original description, this syndrome has been reported in association with asbestosis and silicosis.

Silicosis

Silicosis is a fibrotic disease of the lungs caused by the inhalation of dust containing silicon dioxide. The lung disease resulting from the inhalation of this dust is of three different types:

1. Classical or nodular silicosis.
2. Mixed dust fibrosis.
3. Acute silicosis.

Occupational Exposure to Silica

Since a considerable proportion of the earth's crust consists of silicon dioxide, all forms of underground mining and tunnel construction are associated with possible exposure to silica dust. In addition, significant exposure to silica may occur in a number of other occupations—stonemasonry, sandblasting, foundry work and ceramics.

Incidence and Prevalence

Over the past 30 years, as a result of hygiene measures and substitution of materials, there has been a dramatic decrease in the incidence of silicosis. The number of 'new' cases diagnosed in the UK by the Pneumoconiosis Medical Panels is now low (Table 2).

Pathogenesis

Current hypotheses on the pathogenesis of silicosis are based on animal and cell culture studies, and it is not certain that the conclusions drawn from these studies can be applied to man. The fibrotic process is initiated by lung macrophages when phagocytosis of silica dust occurs, leading to the death and disruption of these cells. The damaged macrophage probably releases various factors which both attract further macrophages to the area and stimulate fibroblasts to fibrogenesis.

Classical (Nodular) Silicosis

Pathology

Dust deposition occurs predominantly in the region of the respiratory bronchioles and the silicotic nodules are found chiefly in this region. The nodule consists of small amounts of dust and large amounts of collagen laid down in a concentric pattern (whorled). As fibrosis progresses, respiratory bronchioles, alveoli and pulmonary vasculature become destroyed.

Clinical Findings

Silicosis, unless complicated by the development of progressive massive fibrosis, tuberculosis or other lung disease, is not usually associated with any symptoms or physical signs. Progressive massive fibrosis develops in about 20 per cent of individuals with classical silicosis and there is a tendency for simple pneumoconiosis to progress, even when exposure to the dust has ceased. When complicated silicosis is present symptoms of progressive dyspnoea develop associated with an unproductive cough. Few physical signs are found, finger clubbing and basal inspiratory crepitations being unusual.

This is the only pneumoconiosis that specifically predisposes to the development of tuberculosis, which should be suspected if the individual develops symptoms of a productive cough, with or without haemoptysis.

Pulmonary Function Tests

In uncomplicated disease no abnormalities of lung function are seen, but occasionally a reduction in vital capacity is observed. In advanced disease a restrictive pattern with reduced lung volumes but only a slight reduction in gas transfer may be found.

Radiology

The radiographic changes of early nodular silicosis consist of small opacities, varying in diameter from 1 mm to 3 mm, present in the upper halves of both lung fields (Figure 4a). These opacities increase in size and number and become distributed throughout the lung fields as the disease progresses. Conglomerate masses (an opacity greater than 1 cm in diameter) may then appear, usually in the upper and mid zones. At an advanced stage these may develop into large, irregular opacities occupying most of the lung fields. Cavitation of these opacities rarely occurs unless the disease is complicated by tuberculosis. Lymph node calcification may occur in silicosis. It occurs in the periphery of the hilar lymph glands (eggshell calcification) (Figure 4b). Evidence of pleural fibrosis may also be seen. Caplan's syndrome occurs in silicosis and the radiographic appearances are indistinguishable from those seen in CWP.

Prognosis

In general, life expectancy is normal in uncomplicated silicosis. However, certain individuals develop progressive disease leading to severe respiratory impairment, cor pulmonale and early death.

Mixed Dust Fibrosis

The condition of mixed dust fibrosis is caused by the inhalation of silica combined with a non-fibrogenic dust, the commonest of which is iron oxide. It has been seen chiefly in haematite miners and in iron and steel foundry workers. The symptoms, physical signs, lung function and radiographic abnormalities of mixed dust fibrosis are similar to those of nodular silicosis. Rarely massive fibrotic lesions may be seen. Mixed dust fibrosis is less often complicated by tuberculosis than is nodular silicosis.

Acute Silicosis

This form of silicosis follows intense exposure, usually of short duration, to silica. The clinical features of the disease are of the rapid development of progressive dyspnoea, cough, sputum and

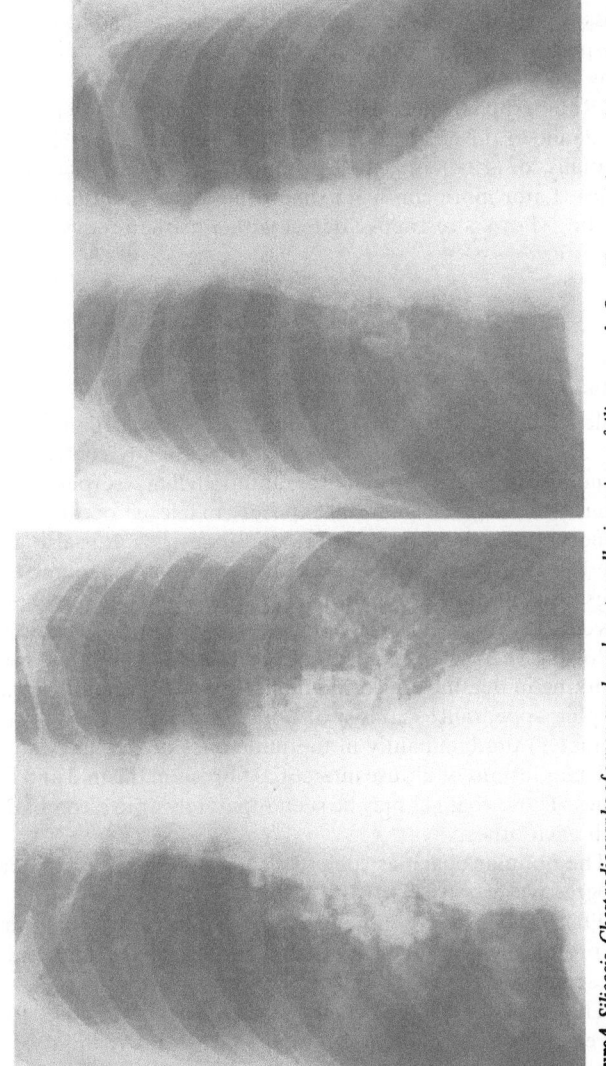

Figure 4. Silicosis. Chest radiographs of a man employed as a tunneller in regions of siliceous rock. Opacities are widespread throughout both lun (1963 ILO category 3; 1977 ILO category 3r). Eggshell calcification of the hilar gland is well seen.

loss of weight. It is a rapidly progressive disease leading to death in respiratory failure. The course of the disease is not influenced by any treatment.

Radiographic appearances resemble those of acute pulmonary oedema or alveolar proteinosis with diffuse lung shadowing, initially of small opacities producing a ground glass appearance. Later more confluent shadowing develops. Lung function testing shows a restrictive defect with a marked reduction in gas transfer.

Other Silicate Pneumoconioses

Talc

Talc is a hydrated magnesium silicate. However, commercial talc, depending on its geographical origin, frequently contains other minerals, including tremolite, anthophyllite, serpentine and quartz. In the past, significant exposure to talc has occurred in talc miners and in the roofing and rubber industries. It is also widely used in the cosmetic, pharmaceutical, paint and ceramic industries. Symptoms of exertional dyspnoea, cough and sputum develop slowly, usually after many years' exposure. Occasionally, following very heavy exposure, the disease may progress rapidly resulting in death from cor pulmonale in a few years. The radiographic appearances consist of nodular opacities (3 to 5 mm in diameter) predominantly in the mid zones of the lungs and the reticular lesions of diffuse interstitial fibrosis in the mid and lower zones. These changes may be seen separately or in a combination with each other.

The nodular opacities coalesce leading to the development of progressive massive fibrosis.

Physical signs are absent except when interstitial fibrosis is present, when finger clubbing and basal crackles may be present.

This type of pneumoconiosis does not predispose to the development of pulmonary tuberculosis. Prevention of talc pneumoconiosis depends on industrial hygiene measures.

Kaolin

Kaolin is a hydrated aluminium silicate. It may cause nodular fibrosis, massive fibrosis and, rarely, diffuse interstitial fibrosis of the lung. The disease only develops after prolonged exposure to high dust concentrations and is therefore seen only in a minority of workers.

Berylliosis

Beryllium is a rare element used in industry for its properties of lightness and strength and its resistance to corrosion and high temperatures. Beryllium has a wide variety of industrial uses, e.g. in non-ferrous alloys, heat resistant ceramics, rocketry and electronic devices. It is absorbed through the lung and skin causing the disease berylliosis in a small proportion of those subjects exposed. Inadvertent exposure to beryllium has occurred in the course of reclamation of non-ferrous alloys, in housewives laundering the clothes of husbands who were in contact with beryllium and in residents living in the neighbourhood of a factory using beryllium.

Two forms of pulmonary disease are recognized: acute and chronic berylliosis.

Acute Berylliosis

Acute berylliosis follows intensive exposure to beryllium and affects the whole of the respiratory tract. The clinical features are those of a chemical pneumonia, occurring within days or, occasionally, weeks of exposure, with the rapid onset of shortness of breath, a cough productive of small quantities of sputum, which may be bloodstained, a tachycardia and inspiratory crepitations over the mid and lower zones of the lungs. The radiographic appearances suggest pulmonary oedema. These abnormalities may take many months to resolve.

The treatment of acute berylliosis includes supplementary oxygen and high dose steroids. About six per cent of these subjects will progress to develop chronic disease.

Chronic Berylliosis

This is a systemic granulomatous disease, predominantly affecting
the lungs and leading to pulmonary fibrosis.

Prevalence. Chronic berylliosis is a rare disease in the UK (Table
2), with only three new cases diagnosed by the Pneumoconiosis
Medical Panels in 1975 and 1976. Berylliosis was not a prescribed
disease in the UK prior to 1974, so accurate estimates of the
incidence of this disease are not available prior to this date.

Pathology. This is characterized by the presence of non-caseating
granulomata found throughout the body including lungs, skin,
lymph glands, liver and spleen. These gramulomata are indistinguishable from those seen in sarcoidosis, extrinsic allergic
alveolitis and Crohn's disease. As the disease progresses,
granulomata become replaced by collagenous tissue producing
the appearances of diffuse interstitial fibrosis in about 50 per cent
of cases.

Pathogenesis. The precise mechanism whereby beryllium produces disease in man is not known, but there are certain features
which suggest that chronic berylliosis is an immunologically
determined disease. Only a small proportion of those exposed to
low concentrations of beryllium will develop disease. A delayed
type skin response may be seen on patch testing with beryllium,
and in the presence of symptomatic disease raised levels of serum
IgG are nearly always found.

Clinical findings. Symptoms are insidious in onset often developing a number of years after only a brief exposure to beryllium. This
latent period is usually less than five years, but has been described
as long as 24 years after the last exposure. The dominant symptoms are of progressive breathlessness accompanied by an unproductive cough. In early disease no abnormal physical signs are
found but, as the disease advances, signs of pulmonary fibrosis
develop. Generalized lymphadenopathy, hepatosplenomegaly,
skin lesions and hypercalcaemia may also be present. The only

features which distinguish berylliosis from sarcoidosis are the absence of ocular, bone and neurological manifestations, a negative Kveim test, normal tuberculin skin reactivity and a positive beryllium patch test. Hilar gland enlargement without evidence of pulmonary disease probably does not occur in berylliosis.

The beryllium patch test (Curtis 1951) when positive only indicates delayed hypersensitivity to beryllium and is not diagnostic of disease. Since the test is not diagnostic, and in addition it has been suggested that the test itself may precipitate an exacerbation of the disease, it is now rarely used.

Pulmonary function tests. The typical changes are entirely nonspecific and are those of diffuse interstitial fibrosis with a restrictive pattern, and a reduction in diffusing capacity. In a small proportion of subjects the restrictive pattern is accompanied by evidence of airways obstruction with a raised residual volume (RV) and RV/TLC (total lung capacity). This is thought to be due to involvement of the small airways by granulomas or fibrosis.

Radiology. The radiographic abnormalities of berylliosis may precede the onset of symptoms by a number of years. Characteristically widespread opacities are present throughout both lung fields, accompanying hilar gland enlargement is uncommon and when present is usually only moderate in degree. The lung opacities vary in size from discrete nodules less than 1 mm in diameter to large confluent shadows.

Treatment. The administration of corticosteroids favourably influences the course of the disease with alleviation of symptoms and prolongation of survival time. In some subjects steroid therapy may result in complete remission, but in many patients long-term maintenance therapy with steroids is required to control symptoms and to prevent progression of the disease.

Further Reading

General

Morgan, K. C. and Seaton, A., *Occupational Lung Diseases*, W. B. Saunders Co., Philadelphia, 1975.

Parkes, W. R., *Occupational Lung Disorders*, Butterworths Ltd, London, 1974.

Asbestos-induced Lung Disease

Becklake, M. R., *American Review of Respiratory Disease*, 1976, **114**, 187.

Coal workers' Pneumoconiosis

Morgan. W. K. C. and Lapp, N. L., *American Review of Respiratory Disease*, 1976, **113**, 531.

2. Sarcoidosis

Ernest Besnier, a renowned Parisian dermatologist, at a clinical meeting in 1889 presented a man who had reddish-purple lesions on his face and arms. Besnier called these lupus pernio. Sir Jonathan Hutchinson of London, between 1889 and 1899, described some cases of a certain skin condition. A Mrs Mortimer had the most conspicuous lesions of these cases and, for a while, the condition was called Mortimer's disease. It is now generally agreed that the description given was that of skin sarcoids.

Boeck of Oslo in 1897 described the clinical and microscopical features of a skin lesion present on various parts of the body of a 36-year-old policeman. Between 1897 and 1915, he described further similar cases and Boeck's name has become associated with the description of skin sarcoids. In later observations, he noted the systemic nature of the disease.

Schaumann of Stockholm in a prize essay on lupus pernio (1914) held, first, that Besnnier's lupus pernio and Boeck's multiple skin sarcoids were manifestations of the same disease and, second, that this disease was systemic in nature. Thus, in sarcoidosis, it was the skin lesions that were first described, and it was mainly due to Boeck and Schaumann that the systemic nature of the condition was established.

Scadding, who has always laid great emphasis on the correct usage of medical terms, suggested the following definition: 'Sarcoidosis is a disease characterized by the presence in *all* of the affected organs of epithelioid cell tubercles without caseation, the older lesions tending to become converted into hyalinized fibrous tissue.' Thus, histological characteristics constitute the basis for diagnosis. Other relevant points are:

1. Epithelioid cell tubercles may also be referred to as sarcoid tubercles or sarcoid granulomata (Plate 1).

2. Aetiology comprises no part of the definition.

3. The absence of caseation in sarcoid tubercles distinguished them from tuberculous tubercles.

4. This definition excludes conditions where sarcoid-like granulomata are found in lymph nodes draining an area which is the site of a malignant tumour, e.g. hilar lymph nodes in the case of bronchial carcinoma and axillary lymph nodes in the case of breast cancer.

In order to understand the origin of epithelioid cells, it is necessary to discuss briefly the mononuclear phagocyte system. (This term replaced the reticuloendothelial system of Aschoff.)

Mononuclear Phagocyte System

Mononuclear phagocytes are derived from precursor cells (promonocytes) in the bone marrow. The mature cells (monocytes) are released into the bloodstream whence they migrate to tissues where they differentiate further into several series of fixed macrophages. Important members of this system are the blood monocytes, Kupffer cells of the liver, histiocytes (reticulum and stellate macrophages) of the spleen and lymph nodes, osteoclasts, alveolar macrophages, and the connective tissue phagocytic cells (tissue histiocytes or macrophages).

The cells of this system are able to remove particulate matter, dyes, carbon particles and partially denatured protein from the bloodstream. Recent work shows that macrophages secrete a number of products locally.

Epithelioid cells of sarcoidosis are derived from these tissue histiocytes or macrophages, and a secretory role is a dominant one of these cells.

Examination of the fine structure of these macrophages in sarcoid tubercles reveals the presence of a deeply indented nucleus, abundant cytoplasm, abundant mitochondria, prominent rough endoplasmic reticulum, numerous electron-dense inclusions and electron-lucent vacuoles.

Giant Cells

Sarcoid tubercles may include giant cells (Plate 2), which are the consequence of:

1. Epithelioid cell aggregation and coalescence.
2. Nuclear division without cytoplasmic division.

The nuclei are placed towards the periphery of the cell and may number 100 or more. In addition to epithelioid and giant cells, lymphocytes are found at the periphery of the sarcoid tubercle.

Three types of inclusions may be found in giant cells: asteroid, conchoidal and crystalline. Asteroid bodies are found within vacuoles and vary in size from small spicules to large star-shaped structures. Conchoidal (or Schaumann) inclusions (Plate 3) are particularly common in lung lesions; they vary in size from $8\,\mu$ to a mass filling the giant cell cytoplasm. These inclusions are comprised partly of calcium and iron salts. Crystalline inclusions are irregular, anisotropic fragments resembling crystals.

Immunology

Probably the best known aspect of immunology is the depression of delayed-type hypersensitivity (T cell inhibition). In sarcoidosis, the tuberculin test is negative in two thirds of the cases. In patients with active sarcoidosis in whom a negative reaction to tuberculin is found and in whom a positive reaction to tuberculin was found prior to the onset of sarcoidosis, the tuberculin reaction, when the disease has resolved, reverts to what it was pre-disease.

Cultured lymphocytes from sarcoidosis patients in whom depression of delayed-type hypersensitivity has been demonstrated react poorly to phytohaemagglutinin (PHA), which normally stimulates lymphocytes to undergo mitosis and blastic transformation.

The reverse situation of T cell inhibition occurs with B lymphocyte activity, shown by increased antibody levels in the blood to herpes simplex, rubella, measles, Epstein–Barr virus and to other viruses.

Circulating immune complexes have been demonstrated in cases of acute sarcoidosis with the combination of bilateral hilar lymphadenopathy and erythema nodosum.

IgE, the main reaginic antibody, is produced and secreted by a numerically small, specific group of plasma cells. The IgE molecules are taken up by special surface receptors on mast cells. The IgE molecules, thus placed with the Fc components attached to these receptors, protrude from the surface of the mast cell and they play an essential part in the pathogenesis of certain common allergic disorders: atopic (extrinsic) asthma, hay fever and eczema. Low or very low levels of IgE in the serum have been found in cases of sarcoidosis.

When a specially prepared extract from selected sarcoid tissue is injected intradermally into patients suffering from active sarcoidosis, in about 75 per cent of the cases a granulomatous sarcoid-like lesion develops, four to six weeks later, at the site of the injection. This is the basis of the Kveim test. A firmly positive reaction can only be established by biopsy of this newly developed lesion.

Clinical Features

Intrathoracic manifestations are, by far, the commonest. Of these, bilateral hilar lymphadenopathy (BHL) is important because it is the commonest single manifestation of the disease.

Bilateral Hilar Lymphadenopathy

BHL usually occurs in patients younger than 30 years, and more frequently in females than in males. In about half of these cases, hilar lymphadenopathy is the only symptom. In about one third of the cases, it is accompanied by erythema nodosum, and in one third of all cases of BHL, a variety of symptoms and signs (including erythema nodosum) may occur in various combinations.

Associated Signs and Symptoms

Arthritis often starts as morning stiffness, sometimes with swelling and local tenderness, in one or both ankles, and spreads to the knees, small joints of the hands, the wrists and elbows. When erythema nodosum occurs in these cases, it usually follows the onset of the arthritis, sometimes by three or four weeks. Sweating, fever and elevated ESR are often found. Rheumatoid factor is usually negative. Joint deformity is not a sequela of the arthritis of early sarcoidosis.

Fever is sometimes prolonged with a temperature up to 39 °C. It may be associated with great listlessness and considerable weight loss.

Subcutaneous nodules are characterized by the development of multiple, mobile, hard, slightly tender nodules on the trunk and limbs. The nodules are often 1 to 1.5 cm in diameter.

Subacute iridocyclitis. Both eyes are more frequently involved than one eye alone. On examination, ciliary congestion and turbidity of aqueous humour are noted. This manifestation may be part of Heerfordt's syndrome (see page 50). Early treatment with local corticosteroid application should be given in all cases of subacute iridocyclitis.

Conjunctival follicles. These may occur with chronic intrathoracic sarcoidosis; palpable nodules are found in the conjunctival folds, especially those of the lower lids. They cause irritation and biopsy shows the presence of typical sarcoid nodules.

Phlyctenular conjunctivitis is an occasional finding and is indistinguishable from that sometimes associated with a primary tuberculous complex in childhood (Phlyctenule (Greek) means a small blister). The vesicles, usually bilateral, occur on the conjunctivae, especially the limbus. A leash of enlarged vessels runs from the corner of the eye to the vesicles. Lacrymation and photophobia may occur. The phlyctenules resolve spontaneously in about two or three weeks' time.

Dry cough may occur, possibly due to pressure of enlarged lymph nodes on the bronchus or to the presence of endobronchial sarcoidosis.

Chest pain may be an important symptom associated with BHL; it may be retrosternal or be sited in either pectoral area. Sometimes, it may be the presenting feature and it may be severe. The cause of the pain is not clear; capsular stretching of lymph nodes and distortion of adjacent structures have been suggested.

Lung mottling, as shown by the PA chest radiograph, indicates the presence of multiple sarcoid tubercles in the lungs. The mottling is bilateral, may be fine or coarse and is usually symmetrical in distribution, although it may be asymmetrical in a minority of cases.

Superficial lymphadenopathy. Enlargement of the cervical nodes, either unilateral or bilateral, may occur. Inguinal nodes may also be enlarged.

Chest Radiographic Appearances with Hilar Lymphadenopathy

On the PA view, the majority of patients show bilateral, symmetrical, moderate enlargement of the hilar lymph nodes. There is usually a well-defined outer border to the abnormal hilar shadow, with a translucent, narrow 'cul de sac' strip between the lower inner aspect of the right hilar shadow and the mediastinal shadow.

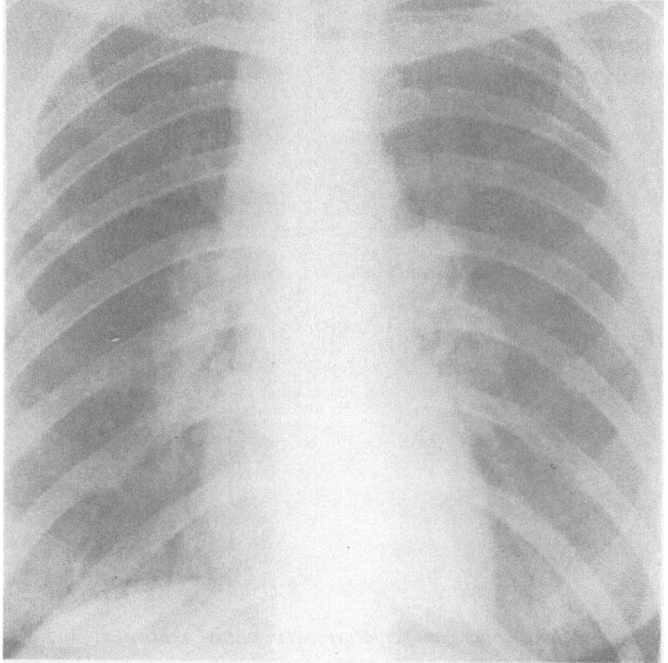

Figure 5. *Bilateral hilar and right paratracheal lymph gland enlargement.*

In about 75 per cent of BHL cases, there is also right paratracheal gland enlargement present, indicated by an extension of the enlarged hilar shadow up to two inches upwards, to the right of the trachea (Figure 5). Lateral chest radiographs and both PA and lateral tomograms confirm the above findings. In a small minority of BHL cases, the enlargement may be gross, simulating the appearances which may be found in Hodgkin's disease (Figure 6).

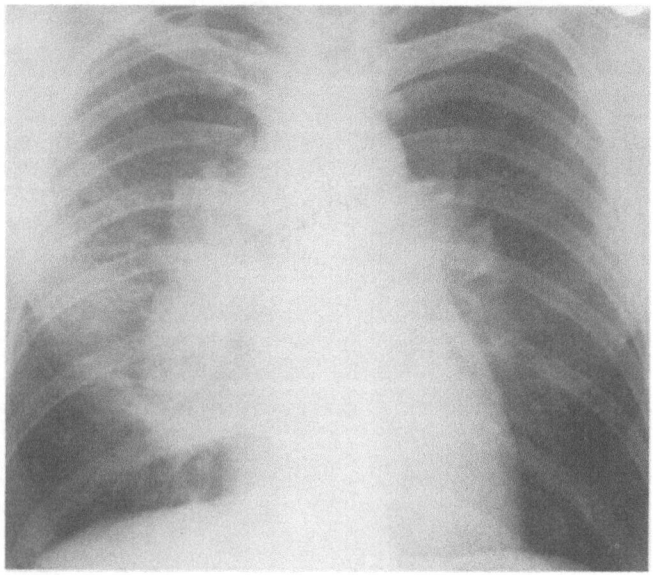

Figure 6. *Massive hilar gland enlargement in a proven case of sarcoidosis.*

In most cases of BHL, the prognosis is good, especially in those cases complicated by erythema nodosum. The glands regress in size and return to normal from three months to two years after the onset of the disease (Figure 7). In the minority of BHL cases which have abnormal lung mottling present on the PA chest radiograph, the lung changes may occur at the time of onset of BHL, or may become evident when a reduction in the size of hilar lymph nodes is being observed. The lung mottling disappears

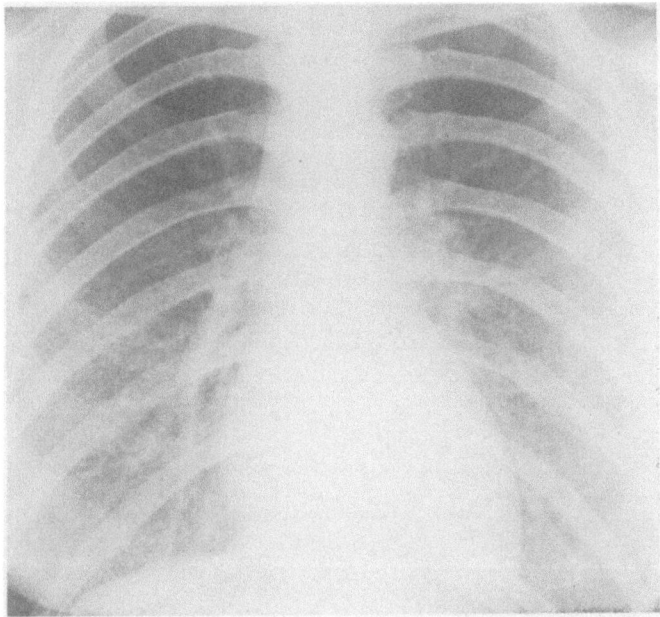

Figure 7. *The same patient as in Figure 5, 20 months later. Gland enlargement has abated and there is miliary shadowing. One year later the chest radiograph was normal.*

in one or two years from the onset of the abnormal lung findings.

In a small minority of BHL cases, the lymph node enlargement does not regress, even after 20 years' observation (Figure 8). In such cases, where histological examination of these permanently enlarged lymph nodes has been possible, an acellular, avascular hyaline fibrosis has been found.

In summary, BHL is the commonest manifestation of sarcoidosis. Regression to normal occurs in the majority of cases.

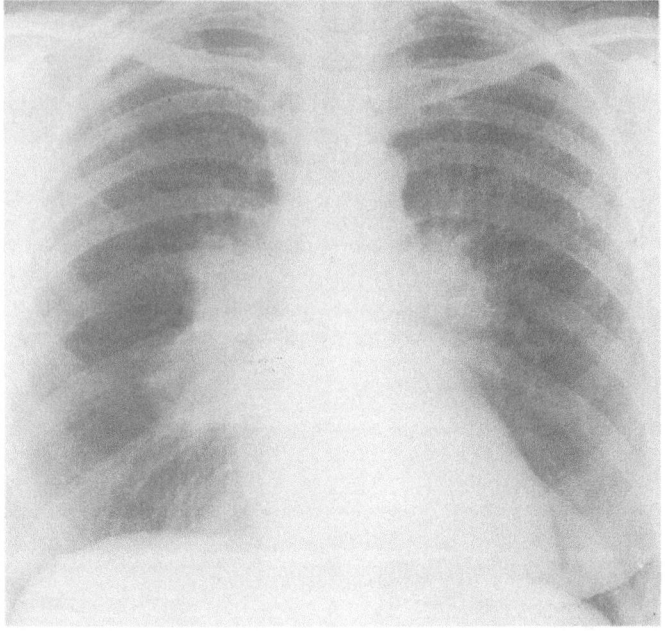

Figure 8. *Bilateral hilar gland enlargement in a proven case of sarcoidosis (1959). There has been no change to the present time.*

Differential Diagnosis of BHL

Tuberculous enlargement of the hilar, paratracheal and other intrathoracic lymph glands may occur in the absence of any radiographic evidence of pulmonary tuberculosis. This is seen particularly in Asian patients. Points in favour of tuberculous disease are:

1. Asymmetry in the lymph node enlargement.

2. Disproportionate enlargement of right paratracheal glands, as compared with the hilar nodes.

3. Positive tuberculin test.

4. Bronchoscopic evidence of a sinus between a major bronchus and an enlarged lymph node.

From material aspirated at the time of bronchoscopy from the region of such sinuses, *Mycobacterium tuberculosis* may be found on direct examination or on culture. However, the differential diagnosis may be difficult. A trial of anti-tuberculous chemotherapy may be of value in reaching the diagnosis.

In Hodgkin's and non-Hodgkin's lymphoma, the lymphatic intrathoracic enlargement may be massive and asymmetrical. Biopsy of a superficial lymph node or of a node removed by mediastinoscopy or at thoracotomy should resolve the problem.

Occasionally in cases of lung cancer, difficulty occurs when a small growth arises in a major bronchus and is associated with bilateral lymph node metastases. Lung cancer occurs in an older age group than sarcoidosis; blood spitting, wheeze, hoarseness (due to left recurrent nerve palsy) and a history of cigarette smoking are important points in favour of lung cancer. In this group of patients bronchoscopy and bronchial biopsy usually reveal the diagnosis.

Pulmonary Sarcoidosis

The lung lesions of sarcoidosis tend to be situated in the region of small lymphatic vessels in the peribronchial, perivascular and subpleural areas.

Individual sarcoid tubercles have only a limited propensity to enlarge. When they become crowded together, as a result of an increase in their number, they show little tendency to fuse (Figure 9).

In subacute sarcoidosis, as already stated, BHL may be accompanied or followed by bilateral lung mottling (Figure 10). Regression of both the BHL and lung mottling occurs in the majority of cases. In other cases, the lung may be involved in sarcoidosis when

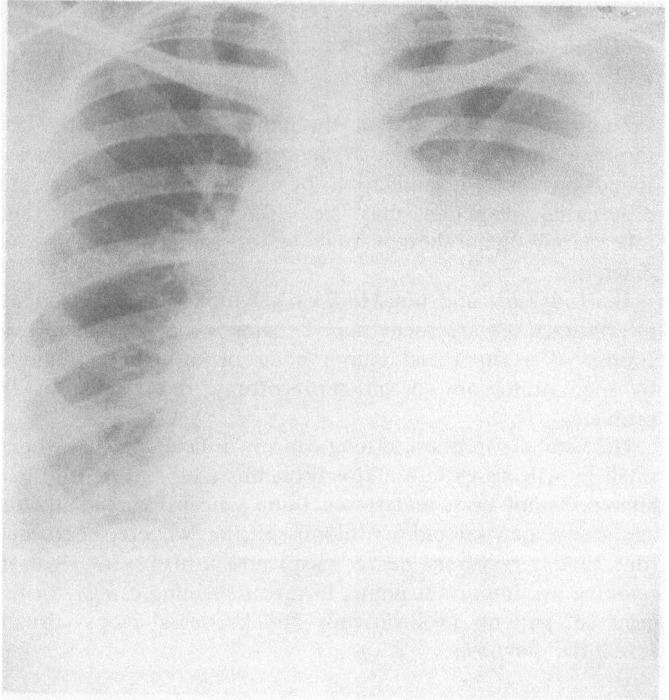

Figure 9. *Large pleural effusion (1). The pleura was studded with sarcoid tubercles.*

there has been no previous history of BHL. These changes are often accompanied by sarcoidosis involving other systems, e.g. skin, bone and superficial lymph nodes. A wide variety of radiographic appearances may be noted:

Figure 10. *(top) Bilateral miliary mottling.*

Figure 11. *(bottom) Coarser shadowing in the right lung. Minor changes in the left lung.*

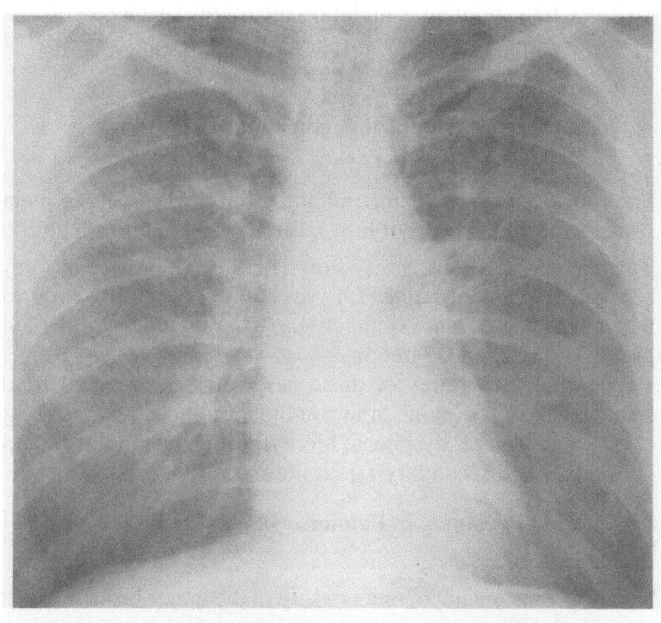

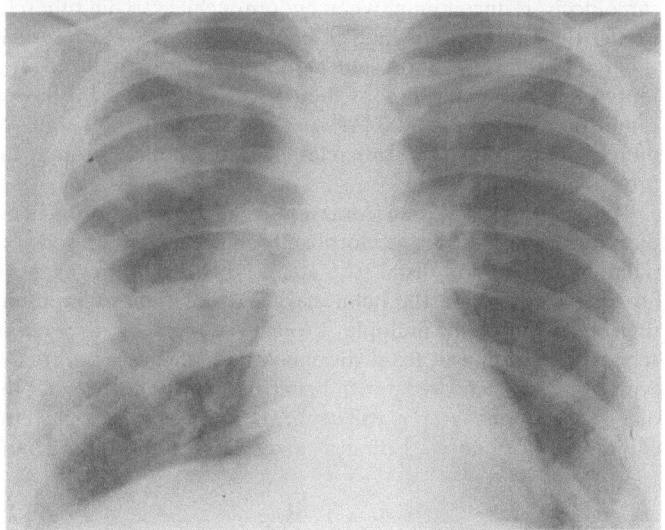

1. Very fine stippling, simulating microlithiasis alveolaris.

2. 'Soft' miliary mottling, resembling miliary tuberculosis.

3. Coarse shadows (Figure 11).

4. Localized, asymmetrical aggregations of mottling.

5. Large masses (Figure 12).

6. Appearances suggesting pulmonary fibrosis and its sequelae: contraction of portions of lungs, bronchiectasis and cavitation.

The history of these cases shows that the lesions may either recover, remain unchanged for years, or develop into a progressive, inexorable advance of the disease to contractions of the lung, bronchiectasis and cavitation.

The clinical features of these cases may be minimal or the following features (alone or in combination) may be seen: cough, chest pain, wheeze, dyspnoea, blood spitting, pneumothorax, cor pulmonale and secondary aspergilloma.

Some Special Features of Pulmonary Sarcoidosis

Bronchostenosis

Significant narrowing of one or more of the major bronchi, due to sarcoidosis, is uncommon; when endobronchial sarcoid tubercles occur, they do not inevitably lead to stenosis—such sarcoid tubercles are probably present more often than is realized. It is more likely that these lesions themselves cause bronchostenosis rather than by the external pressure of enlarged lymph nodes or direct spread of sarcoid tubercles from the nodes through the bronchial wall.

The symptoms resulting from stenoses of the major bronchi are dyspnoea, wheeze (may be localized) and recurrent episodes of pulmonary infection distal to a stenosis. Difficulty in diagnosis arises in cases where the pulmonary sarcoidosis has waxed and then resolved with multiple bronchostenoses as the major sequelae, resulting in fixed dyspnoea and wheeze as obtrusive symptoms. Bronchoscopy with bronchial biopsy may reveal the diagnosis. Bronchography will confirm the presence and show the extent of the stenoses. Either as a result of repeated infection,

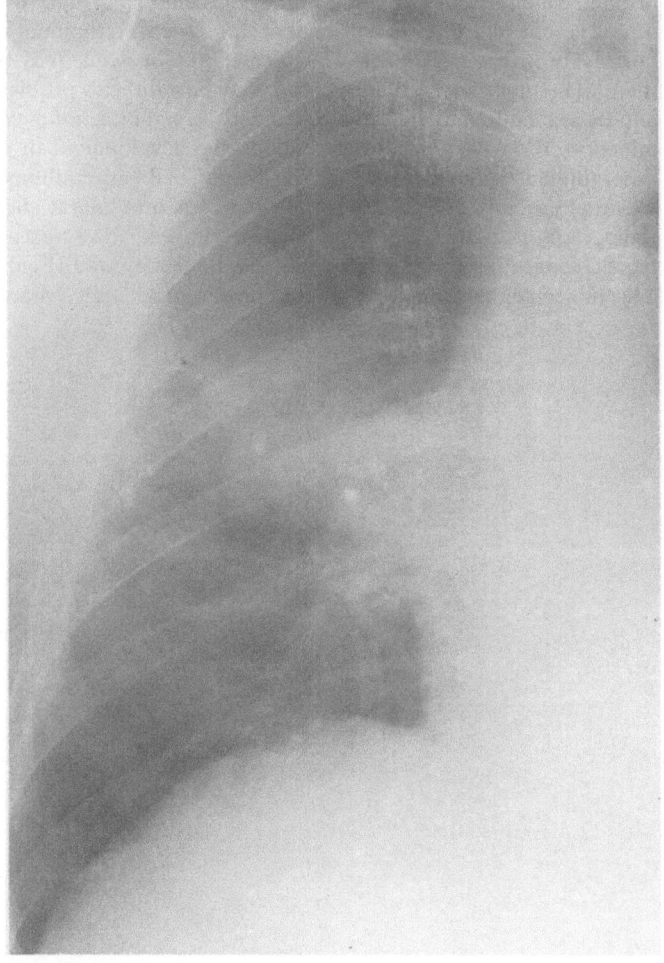

Figure 12. *Mass in the right lung. Sarcoid tissue was proven on biopsy.*

　　　　　　　　Interstitial Lung Disease

distal to a stenosis, or as a result of the contraction and distortion of a segment of a lobe(s) consequent upon the development of fibrosis, bronchiectasis, thick-walled cavitation or bullae may be found. Haemoptyses, often repeated, may be a difficult problem and occasionally may be fatal. Secondary *Aspergillus fumigatus* infection in a cavity wall often leads to the development of an aspergilloma within the cavity. The fungus ball (aspergilloma) eventually nearly fills the cavity; on both PA and lateral chest radiographs it appears as a dense shadow with a narrow–crescentic slit, separating the aspergilloma from the cavity wall (Figure 13). In such circumstances, repeated haemoptyses are common,

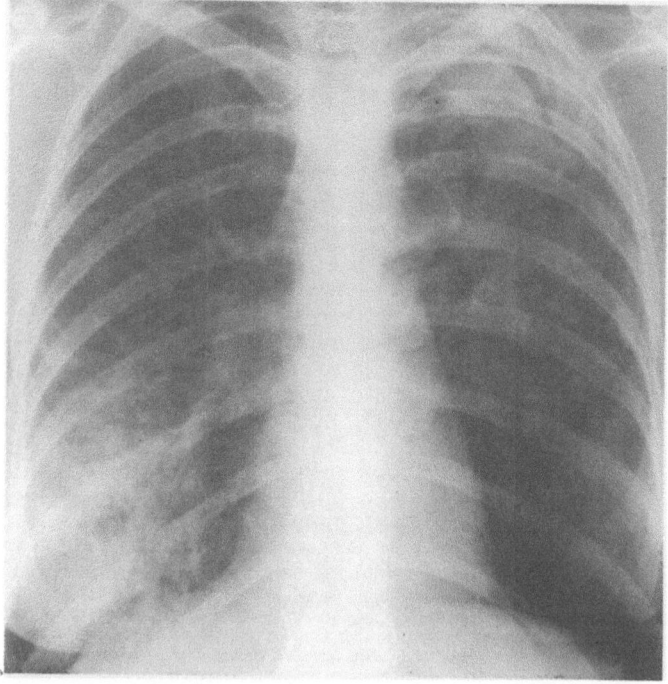

Figure 13. *Aspergilloma in cavity, left upper lobe, in a patient with extensive pulmonary sarcoidosis.*

often troublesome and occasionally necessitate a lobectomy. Positive precipitins against *A. fumigatus* are found in the serum of patients with secondary aspergilloma—the precipitin test usually indicates that a number of antigens present in *A. fumigatus* are involved.

Pleurisy

A number of recent reports indicate that pleural involvement in sarcoidosis is commoner than has been recognized hitherto. In these cases, sarcoid tubercles are present on the pleural surface and tend to bulge from it. Clinically, there may be pleural pain, pleural effusion (sometimes massive), or thickened pleura present. Pleurisy is always associated with the presence of sarcoid tubercles elsewhere in the lungs. It seems to occur most frequently in women of African ancestry.

Calcifications

Scadding (1961) drew attention to the development of calcification in lymph nodes involved in sarcoidosis. It occurs in the avascular acellular hyaline tissue which is a sequela of sarcoid tubercles (occasionally intrapulmonary calcification may also be found in these cases).

Hilar, mediastinal and supraclavicular groups of lymph nodes may be involved in this change. Chest radiographs show that the calcification is both bilateral and symmetrical.

In contrast, calcification in tuberculous lymph nodes tends to be unilateral, often with a marked change in the paratracheal glands.

This type of calcification in sarcoidosis is unrelated to the calcium metabolic abnormalities found in this disease.

Differential Diagnosis of Pulmonary Sarcoidosis

Only some of the many conditions which may give rise to diffuse bilateral lung abnormalities will be considered here.

Pulmonary Tuberculosis

Pulmonary tuberculosis more often affects upper and posterior segments than lower and anterior ones. However, in some cases of

chronic progressive pulmonary sarcoidosis, the PA chest radiographic appearances may be indistinguishable from those of
tuberculosis (Figures 14 and 15), where examination of sputum,

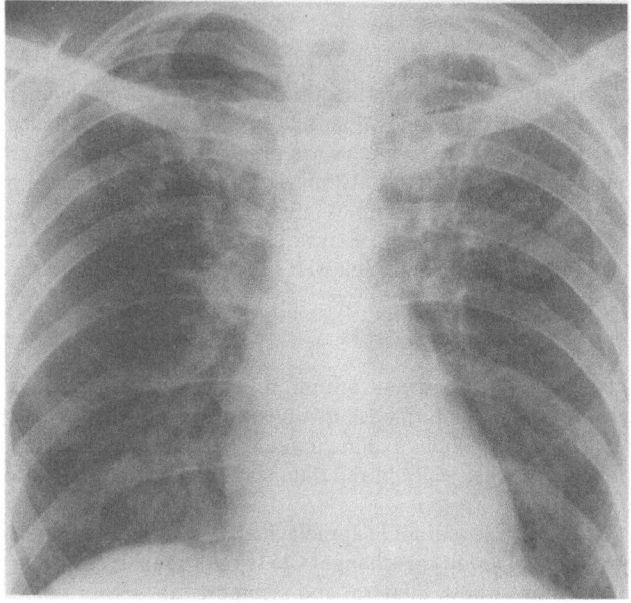

Figure 14. *The appearances simulate tuberculosis.*

either directly or by culture, may reveal the presence of *M.
tuberculosis*. In addition, in cases of active pulmonary
tuberculosis, the tuberculin test is strongly positive in most cases
and the symptoms may comprise cough, purulent odourless
sputum, haemoptyses, weight loss, fever, night sweats and frequently lassitude and listlessness.

Pulmonary sarcoidosis and tuberculosis may coexist or the
one may follow the other, compounding the difficulties in
diagnosis.

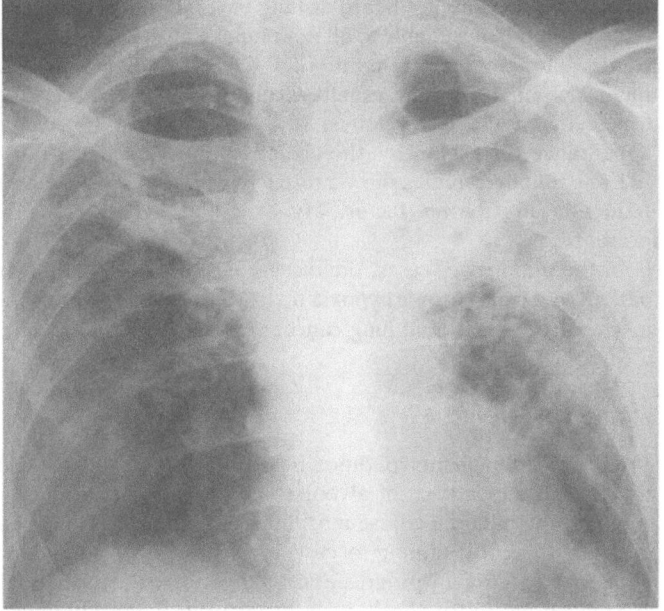

Figure 15. *The same patient as in Figure 14, four years later. The patient died from massive haemoptysis. The radiograph shows sarcoidosis with fibrosis, bronchostenoses and cavity formation in both lungs.*

Industrial Disease

Industrial disease, e.g. coalminer's pneumoconiosis, may be present. Here, a full industrial history is important. Often, in such cases, previous chest radiographs may exist.

Interstitial Pneumonia

Interstitial pneumonia (fibrosing alveolitis) is a condition occurring mainly in middle-aged and elderly persons. It is characterized by increasing shortwindedness, tachypnoea, dry irritating cough, usually finger and toe clubbing and rarely by hypertrophic osteoarthropathy. On auscultation (in most cases) showers of fine inspiratory crackles are heard at lung bases. Patients often complain of their being unable to fill their lungs fully with a feeling of a sudden stop to their inspiration. PA chest radiographs show increased bilateral and usually symmetrical linear markings, especially in the lower lobes, sometimes with a honeycomb appearance (in a minority, the changes are asymmetrical).

Lung function studies show a restrictive pattern, with a marked reduction in transfer factor. Hypoxia and hypocapnoea are present.

In the majority of cases, the disease is slowly progressive and patients die from chronic hypoxia up to 15 years after the onset. A few die from associated lung cancer.

Diffuse Malignant Disease

Primary: Although this condition is very uncommon, the PA chest radiograph appearance of alveolar cell cancer of the lung may simulate the bilateral coarse mottling of sarcoidosis. This apparently multicentric tumour occurs in middle aged and elderly persons, and it usually progresses relentlessly to death by hypoxia. A small minority of these cases expectorate large volumes of watery sputum, up to 500 ml/24 hours or more. Cytological examination of the sputum may reveal the presence of malignant cells.

Metastases

When the general condition of a patient remains good and there are few symptoms, the presence of multiple lung metastases may pose great difficulty in diagnosis—chest radiographic appearances vary from fine miliary mottling to bilateral coarse nodules. As with sarcoidosis, these appearances may remain unchanged for years, although usually repeated careful examination over a period of months resolves the problem. Thyroid, ovary, testis and gastrointestinal tract are the commoner sites for primary growths in such circumstances.

Lymphangitis Carcinomatosa

In lymphangitis carcinomatosa there is a retrograde spread of malignant tissue, from metastases in hilar lymph nodes, along the lymphatic vessels of the lung to the pleura, where a diffuse interweaving of mosaic lymphatic vessels stuffed with malignant tissue may be seen at postmorten examination.

The condition involves both lungs (occasionally serial chest radiographs reveal that the changes involve one lung before the other).

Clinical features of lymphangitis carcinomatosa are an inexorably increasing shortness of breath, cough, tachypnoea, sometimes wheeze and often pleural effusion. The clinical history is usually of short duration and the presence of a primary growth may already be known. Common sites for such primaries are the gastrointestinal tract (including pancreas), breast, ovary and the lung itself. In the breast cancer cases, lymphangitis carcinomatosa may not develop for a decade or more after a mastectomy. Chest radiographs reveal an increase in the linear lung markings and the mediastinal lymph nodes may appear enlarged. There may be an associated leucoerythroblastic anaemia.

Histiocytosis X (Eosinophilic Granuloma)

Histiocytosis is uncommon and of unknown aetiology. It occurs mainly in young adults and is manifest on the PA chest radiograph as diffuse lung shadowings, linear and mottled, leading to extensive honeycombing of the lungs with severe pulmonary disability and a tendency to develop pneumothoraces. There may be associated multiple lytic bone lesions in the skull or long bones.

Bronchopulmonary Aspergillosis

The chest radiograph appearances of bronchopulmonary aspergillosis may, in its advanced stages, simulate some cases of chronic progressive pulmonary sarcoidosis, i.e. bilateral upper lobe contraction with bronchiectasis and cavitation.

Patients suffering from bronchopulmonary aspergillosis are atopic and also suffer from bronchial asthma. In addition, chest radiographs may show recurrent pulmonary infiltrates in different lung segments. Also, a type III (Coombs and Gell) hypersensitivity reaction (immune complex deposition) may cause damage to the walls of the bronchi, more especially in the medium-sized bronchi.

Positive skin tests for *Aspergillus fumigatus* and a positive test for the presence in the serum of precipitins against *Aspergillus fumigatus* are found in these cases.

Ankylosing Spondylitis

In a minority of cases of ankylosing spondylitis, upper lobe changes, as shown by the chest radiograph may simulate chronic sarcoidosis. A clinical history of low back pain and stiffness made worse by rest, painful heels, tender areas on ribs and tuber ischii and the characteristic radiographic changes of the spine and sacroiliac joints should establish the diagnosis.

Heerfordt's Syndrome

One variety of extensive active sarcoidosis is Heerfordt's syndrome. This comprises salivary gland enlargement due to sarcoid tubercle infiltration—the parotid gland is most frequently involved. The enlargement is usually bilateral, reaching maximal size in one or two weeks; one gland may enlarge two to three weeks before the other. Less frequently, the submandibular, lingual and minor salivary glands are involved (normal appearance of lip mucosa may be found where the minor glands of the same mucosa are affected by sarcoidosis). Dryness of the mouth may be a symptom.

Facial nerve palsy is also found and is unilateral more often than bilateral. Palsy frequently occurs with enlargement of the ipsilateral parotid gland.

Iridocyclitis may occur (see page 33).

Enlarged lacrymal glands may be palpated or seen by lifting the upper eyelid. Dryness of the eyes may be a symptom. The full syndrome is uncommon. Associated sarcoidosis in lungs, lymph nodes and skin is common.

Skin Sarcoids

Approximately 15 per cent of cases of sarcoidosis develop sarcoid tubercles in the skin, either at presentation or during the course of the disease.

Lupus Pernio

Lupus pernio consists of chilblain-like swellings affecting, singly or in combination, the face, fingers and toes. It develops slowly. On the face it may be disfiguring, involving the nose and cheeks and sometimes forehead and ears. The lesions are purple–red, shiny and firm. When lupus pernio involves the fingers or toes, the underlying phalanx is usually affected by sarcoidosis. The radio-

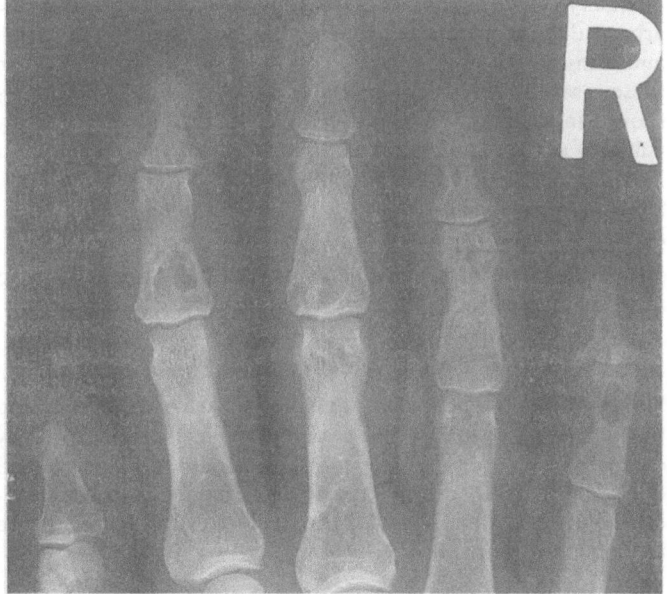

Figure 16. *Characteristic cystic bone changes. This patient had lupus pernio on his face and fingers.*

graphic appearances of bone sarcoid are described on page 56—reticular (lattice-like) rarefactions are especially seen in these cases (Figure 16). About half of lupus pernio cases have associated skin sarcoids (large and small) and persistent lung changes which proceed to pulmonary fibrosis in most cases.

Papules and Plaques

The other skin sarcoids present a wide range of manifestations, mainly papules and plaques. The lesions are usually multiple, firm and often extend further than inspection might indicate. The entire cutis is affected, with an intact epidermis.

The outer border of the lesion is raised and the centre tends to heal. The colour of the lesion varies from faint red to purple or brown with a fine superficial desquamation. The lesions of the plaque type have a predilection for the face, outer aspects of the arms and the shoulders. One uncommon type, found on the trunk and arms, is the deep cutaneous sarcoid of Darier–Roussy. In these cases the lesions are inconspicuous, the overlying skin may show a faint dusky red or purple line, but the lesions are easily palpable as firm nodules attached to the skin.

Subcutaneous Nodules

Subcutaneous nodules often accompany bilateral hilar lymphadenopathy with erythema nodosum. The nodules tend to resolve along with the BHL.

Scar Infiltrations

Scar infiltrations tend to occur at an early stage of the disease and their course follows that of the concomitant lung sarcoidosis. They consist of single or multiple purple nodules which develop in operation or injury scars. A particular example is the development of sarcoid granulomata at the site of previous venepuncture in blood donors.

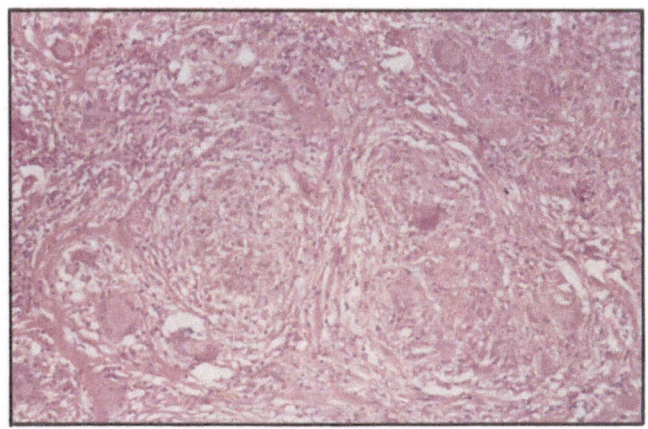

Plate 1. *Lung. The alveolar pattern is obliterated by granulomata contain-ing epithelioid cells and some giant cells. (Courtesy of Dr K. V. Lodge.)*

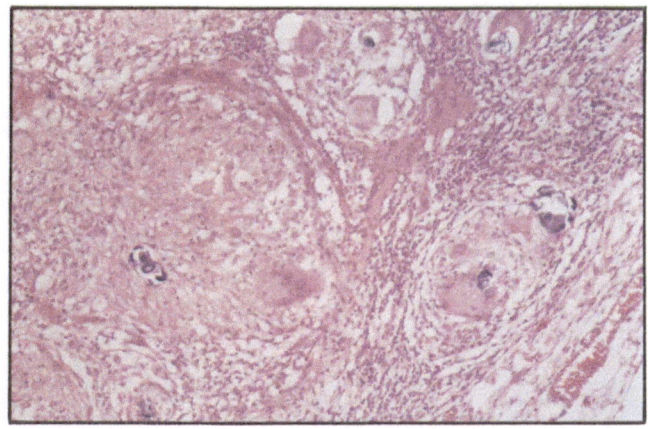

Plate 2. *Lung. Epithelioid foci with giant cells and Schaumann bodies. (Courtesy of Dr K. V. Lodge).*

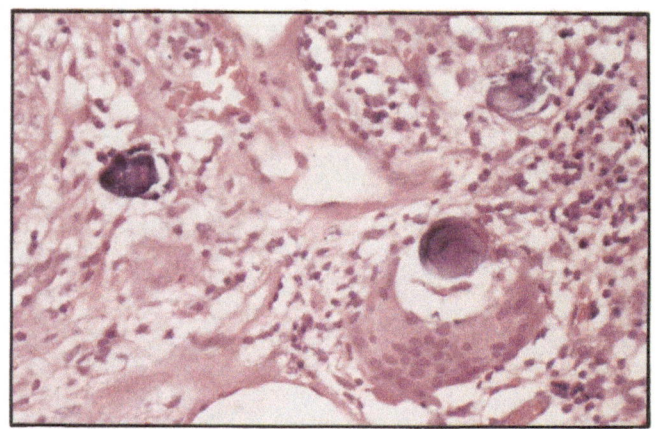

Plate 3. *Lung. Higher power view of Plate 2 showing Schaumann bodies. (Courtesy of Dr K. V. Lodge.)*

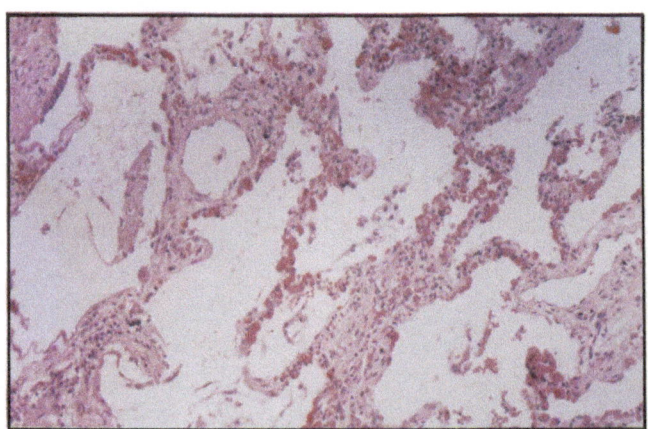

Plate 4. *Cryptogenic fibrosing alveolitis. Marked thickening and distortion of the alveolar network. Very few cells are seen in the alveolar spaces.*

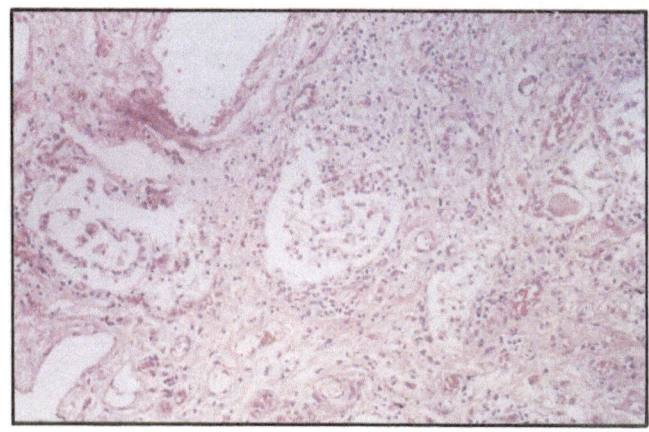

Plate 5. *Cryptogenic fibrosing alveolitis. Advanced stage with destruction of the alveoli, those remaining containing mononuclear-like cells.*

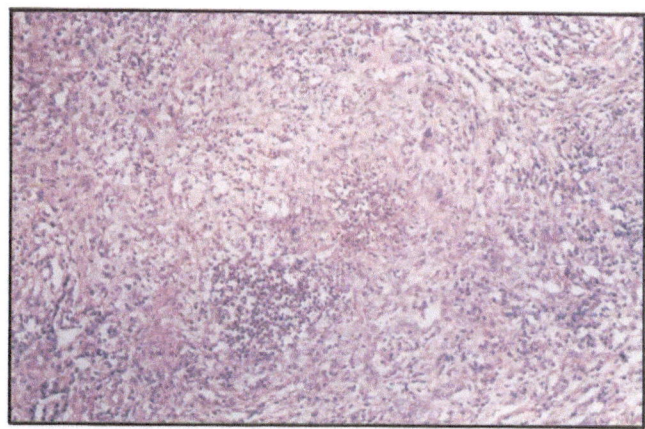

Plate 6. *Wegener's granulomatosis. Intense cellular reaction with necrosis, giant cell formation and eosinophil infiltration.*

Heart Sarcoidosis

Heart sarcoidosis is uncommon, but should be considered when patients with proven sarcoidosis develop an arrhythmia, a conduction defect or congestive heart failure. The myocardium is affected most, whereas valvular and pericardial involvement are rare.

The myocardial lesions have the following characteristics:

1. Have a patchy distribution and, at postmortem examination, the appearances to the naked eye may resemble those of ischaemic fibrosis.

2. May involve the right ventricle and the atria, as well as the left ventricle.

3. Have a special propensity to involve the upper parts of the ventricular septum.

Clinical Features

The commonest features are rhythm disturbances, including complete heart block, ventricular tachycardia, multifocal ventricular premature systoles, atrial fibrillation and atrial flutter. Persistent hypotension may be a feature and unexpected or sudden death may occur. Congestive heart failure due to diffuse myocardial disease may occur, particularly in the 35 to 60 year age group.

Most authors suggest that steroid therapy should be given when myocardial sarcoidosis is suspected.

Chronic cor pulmonale may occur in patients suffering from chronic pulmonary sarcoidosis. In some patients this is due to compression and/or invasion of branches of the pulmonary artery by sarcoid tissues. In others, co-existing chronic bronchitis is the major factor.

Nervous System Involvement

Involvement of the nervous system by sarcoidosis occurs in about five per cent of cases. Sarcoid tubercles, infiltrating the basal meninges, probably cause most of the symptoms. The meninges are found to be thickened and opaque. Clinically, the cranial nerves, meninges and hypothalamus (with pituitary) are the most frequently affected parts of the nervous system.

Cranial Nerve Involvement

Cranial nerve involvement, either of one or many nerves, tends to occur early in the disease. The facial and optic nerves are the two most frequently affected. Facial nerve palsy occurs unilaterally more often than bilaterally. In some cases it may be associated with parotid gland enlargement due to sarcoidosis, resulting in nerve compression. In others, the temporal relationship between the parotid enlargement and the facial palsy excludes this cause. Sense of taste may or may not be lost on the affected side. Resolution of the facial palsy may be incomplete.

Optic Nerve Involvement

Blurring of vision, papilloedema and the presence of sarcoid tubercles on the retinae are important features of optic nerve involvement. Both facial and optic nerve involvement may occur alone. However, Matthews (1959) has pointed out a recognizable clinical syndrome of fluctuating asymmetrical multiple cranial nerve lesions. This occurs in the subacute, remittent forms of sarcoidosis where bilateral hilar lymphadenopathy, erythema nodosum, iritis and parotid gland enlargement may be found. Associated findings, indicating that other parts of the nervous system may be involved in these cases, are large areas of hypaegesia (with pain) on the trunk.

Direct involvement of the cranial nerves or meninges is the likely cause of this syndrome. In the most chronic forms of sarcoidosis basal meningitis due to infiltration by sarcoid tubercles may give rise to abnormal mental states, headaches, cranial nerve pareses, ataxia, grand mal, focal fits, hypersomnia, hypothermia, diabetes insipidus, aphasia, nerve deafness and anterior pituitary failure.

When the granulomatous change in the meninges forms a mass, then symptoms of a space-occupying intracranial lesion may occur.

Calcium Metabolism in Sarcoidosis

For about 30 years it has been known that in a small minority of sarcoidosis cases hypercalcaemia and hypercalciuria may be found. The related symptoms include thirst, polyuria, anorexia, nausea, weight loss, lassitude, irritability and mental depression. These features may be the presenting ones and may dominate the clinical picture.

Special points in the clinical assessment of these cases are the presence of:

1. Corneal deposits called band keratopathy.

2. Calcium deposits in the skin.

3. Renal disturbances, with or without nephrocalcinosis, leading to renal failure.

Recently, abnormalities of calcium metabolism in normocalcaemic sarcoidosis cases were found to be common, including increased calcium absorption by the bowel, hypercalciuria and increased bone turnover.

The cause of these abnormalities remains obscure. Recently, however, a case of sarcoidosis has been reported in which hypercalcaemia was associated with abnormally high circulating levels of 1, 25-dihydroxycholecalciferol, the active hormonal metabolite of vitamin D. It was suggested that the hypercalcaemia was due to a defect in the regulation or production of this hormone (Papapoulos et al. 1979).

In only a small minority of sarcoidosis patients with calcium abnormalities is hypercalcaemia found, and hypercalcaemia might be termed 'the tip of the iceberg' in these abnormalities. The evidence does not confirm higher serum calcium levels in the summer months in these cases.

The natural history of calcium metabolic abnormalities in sarcoidosis has not been well elucidated. This is in part due to the use of corticosteroids in treating hypercalcaemic cases, when the serum calcium levels return to normal after corticosteroid use. None the less, the evidence is that the disturbance is of short duration.

Renal involvement in sarcoidosis has the following features:

1. Hypercalcaemia (already mentioned).

2. Sarcoid nephropathy. This is independent of hypercalcaemia, and occurs infrequently. Massive renal changes due to presence of sarcoid tubercles are very uncommon, but, when present, are characterized by proteinuria, azotaemia, urinary casts and haematuria.

Renal biopsy will reveal the familiar tubercles of sarcoidosis.

Bone Sarcoidosis

Changes in bone due to the presence of sarcoid tubercles are uncommon and are mainly found in chronic sarcoidosis especially with lupus pernio and other skin sarcoids. Most cases have evidence of intrathoracic sarcoidosis present as well.

Neville et al. (1977) in a series of 29 cases of bone sarcoidosis divided the cases into three groups:

1. Lytic—punched-out cysts.

2. Permeative—'tunnelling' of cortical bone leading to a change in the architecture of the bone, resulting in a reticular pattern on the bone radiographs.

3. Destructive—with deformity, fracture and sequestration, as sequelae.

Soft tissue swelling may occur over bone sarcoid cysts. The bones most frequently affected are the proximal and middle finger phalanges and the heads of the metacarpals; toe phalanges and metatarsals may also be involved.

When lupus pernio and bone sarcoidosis are associated (Figure 16) the skin over an affected bone is often the site of lupus pernio.

Liver Sarcoidosis

Biopsy studies have shown that, in nearly two thirds of all cases of sarcoidosis, sarcoid tubercules are found to be present in the liver and that sarcoidosis is probably the commonest cause of multiple liver granulomata.

In the majority of cases where sarcoid tubercles have been found in the liver, there are no symptoms associated with these lesions. In a small minority, however, a clinical picture may emerge, where progressive destruction of the bile canaliculi by sarcoid tubercles occurs. Fibrosis follows and the picture resembles primary biliary cirrhosis with jaundice, pruritus and high serum alkaline phosphatase levels, but with negative tests for presence of serum antimitochondrial antibodies. The condition has been referred to as chronic intrahepatic cholestasis of sarcoidosis. It occurs particularly in young male Negroes in the USA. Gall bladder involvement and biliary tract obstruction due to sarcoidosis have also been reported.

Spleen Involvement

The incidence of splenic involvement is not clear, but in fatal cases of sarcoidosis, the spleen is involved in the great majority. Even in fatal cases, the spleen is only palpable in a minority and enlargement is rarely massive.

Associated anaemia, leucopenia or thrombocytopenia have all been described in association with splenic involvement with sarcoidosis. Splenectomy may be followed by a return to normal blood findings.

Biochemistry

Although the epithelial cells and giant cells found in sarcoid tubercles are derived from tissue histiocytes (macrophages), which are members of the monocytic phagocyte system, their secretory role is important.

One enzyme which is secreted mainly by monocytes and polymorphonuclear leucocytes is lysozyme. It is, therefore, understandable that due to their tissue histiocyte (macrophage) origin, epithelioid cell activity may be associated with an elevated level of this enzyme. This has been found in active sarcoidosis and the rise in this serum enzyme level is an index of the total mass of sarcoid tubercles present. It is probably most useful when serial estimations are made, thereby assessing progression or regression of the disease.

A second enzyme secreted by sarcoid tubercles is the serum angiotensin converting enzyme (ACE). Angiotensin I, a decapeptide, is produced in the liver and is metabolically inactive. ACE cleaves off a dipeptide (histidyl–leucine) to produce the vasoactive octapeptide, Angiotensin II. ACE is known to exist normally in high concentrations in the lung. It is bound to the surface membranes of endothelial cells of the pulmonary capillaries. High levels of ACE have been found in active sarcoidosis, whereas no such elevation was found in other diffuse lung conditions, e.g. bronchiectasis, tuberculosis, lung cancer and chronic bronchitis. Estimation of ACE should be of value in corroborating a diagnosis of active sarcoidosis; and, when performed serially, in assessing the progression or regression of the disease with or without treatment.

Aetiology

At present, the aetiology of sarcoidosis remains obscure. However, several theories have been propounded. Probably the most controversial one deals with the relationship between sarcoidosis and mycobacterial infection. It is known that infection with *M. tuberculosis* and sarcoidosis may coexist; sarcoidosis may closely precede or may closely follow tuberculosis, and sarcoidosis may follow close contact with infectious tuberculosis. In addition, although there are some differences, the histological appearances in both diseases have many similarities.

The most widely accepted theory relating these two diseases is that sarcoidosis is the result of infection by *M. tuberculosis* in a patient whose tissue responses to the presence of those organisms are peculiar, e.g. non-caseating tubercles against caseating tubercles, and negative or weakly positive tuberculin tests against strongly positive ones.

Arguments against this theory state that it is not possible, in general, to grow *M. tuberculosis* from sarcoid tissue; that sarcoidosis is not influenced by antituberculous chemotherapy; that in some countries, a divergent incidence of sarcoidosis and tuberculosis has been noted. Interest in this theory has been reinforced by work carried out by Mitchell (1976), who was able to passage repeatedly an agent obtained from sarcoid tissue. The true nature of this agent is not clear—it might be a protoplast form of *M. tuberculosis*, persisting as an intracellular parasite of connective tissue cells.

Epidemiological evidence has been adduced of an apparent correlation between the birth places of sarcoidosis patients and the distribution of pine forests.

Pine pollen contains diaminopimelic acid which also occurs in sarcoid tissue and mycobacteria. Pine pollen, when introduced into some experimental animals, can produce sarcoid-like tubercles. However, sarcoidosis occurs in countries where there are no pine forests.

Although mycobacteria and pine pollen may be causal factors in some cases of sarcoidosis, for the majority of cases at present the issue must be left open.

Epidemiology

Sarcoidosis has a world wide distribution. Acute sarcoidosis occurs most frequently in young adults, and the less common chronic progressive sarcoidosis occurs in the 30 to 60 year age group.

Sarcoidosis may occur in childhood, where the variety of presenting symptoms may make the diagnosis difficult. The Irish in Britain have a higher incidence than the rest of the population. In the USA, the frequency of sarcoidosis is much higher in the Negro than in the white population, and tends to be florid in its manifestations in the Negro population.

As some people may develop sarcoidosis with only a few unobtrusive symptoms and subsequently go on to complete resolution, it is likely that many cases go by undiagnosed to full recovery.

Diagnosis

As the definition of sarcoidosis hinges on finding a certain histological change in all tissues examined, it is clear that biopsy of one, or preferably more than one, tissue is important, e.g. superficial lymph nodes, skin lesions, nodules in old scars and liver. In conjunction with fibreoptic bronchoscopy, biopsies may be of great help in demonstrating endobronchial and lung sarcoid tubercles, especially in cases of BHL.

Biopsies may also be taken from lip mucosa (for minor salivary gland involvement), muscle and nasal mucosa.

The Kveim–Siltzbach skin test tends to be positive in the early active cases, e.g. BHL, and negative in the chronic progressive cases.

The commonest single presentation of sarcoidosis is BHL, often with erythema nodosum and polyarthritis (occurring together or alone). When this occurs, especially in young persons, it is reasonable to make a diagnosis on the clinical findings alone.

A difficult problem arises when the presence of diffuse lung changes is indicated by the chest radiograph and where there is no evidence of BHL, past or present, or evidence of extrathoracic sarcoidosis. In such cases, the Kviem–Siltzbach test may be negative and drill biopsy or open lung biopsy should be considered. Advantages of open lung biopsy are that the lung can be inspected, the biopsy site can be carefully selected, and lymph node and liver biopsy can be carried out at the same time. The disadvantages are the discomfort and the risk of this procedure to the patient.

In two thirds of sarcoid cases, the tuberculin test is negative and in the remainder of cases severe reactions are not found.

ACE, where reliable facilities are available for its estimation in serum, should prove of value both in diagnosis and in assessing the changing activity of the total mass of sarcoid tubercles present.

Treatment

Sarcoidosis, in most cases, is a self-limiting illness, and in these cases there is no indication for treatment.

Prednisolone, which suppresses the disease, is the mainstay of treatment, when indicated. It does *not* cure the disease. There are clear indications for its use in:

1. Eye sarcoidosis, e.g. iridocyclitis. Prednisolone is given to prevent permanent damage to vision.

2. Hypercalcaemia. A small dose may be sufficient to reduce the serum calcium levels to within normal limits. Calcium metabolic disorders in sarcoidosis are self-limiting, thus, prednisolone therapy will be needed for a short period, perhaps six months.

3. Myocardial sarcoidosis—Presumably prednisolone minimizes the incidence of serious arrhythmias.

The indications for prednisolone therapy in pulmonary sarcoidosis are less clearly defined. There is no doubt that prednisolone will suppress the pulmonary changes as indicated by the radiographic appearances. Commonly used criteria for its use are deterioration in pulmonary function and progression of the radiographic changes after 9 to 12 months' surveillance. A common dosage in these cases is 15 mg prednisolone daily.

References

Matthews, W. B., *J. Neurol. Neurosurg. Psychiat.*, 1965, **28**, 23.

Mitchell, D. N., *Ann. N.Y. Acad. Sci.*, 1976, **278**, 233.

Mitchell, D. N., Rees, R. J. and Goswani, K. K., *Lancet,* 1976, **ii**, 761.

Neville, E., Carstairs, L. S. and James, G. D., *Q.J.Med.*, 1977, **xlvi**, 215.

Papapoulas, S. H., Clemens, T. L., Fraher, L. J., Lewin, I. G., Sandler, I. M. and O'Riordan, J. L. M., *Lancet,* 1979, **i**, 627.

Scadding, J. G., *Sarcoidosis,* Eyre and Spottiswoode, London, 1967.

Further Reading

Mononuclear Phagocyte System

Hobart, M. J. and McConnell, I., *The Immune System,* Blackwell Scientific Publications, London, 1975, Ch. 12.

Immunology and Ultrastructure

Carr, I. and Norris, P., *J. Path.,* 1977, **122,** 29.

James, G. D., Neville, E. and Walker, A., *Am.J.Med.,* 1975, **59,** 388.

Hedfors, E. and Norberg, R., *Clin.Exp.Immunol.,* 1974, **16,** 493.

Yagura, T., Shimizu, M., Yamamura, Y. and Tachibana, T., *Clin.Exp.Immunol.,* 1975, **21,** 289.

Calcium Disturbances

Reiner, M., Sigurdsson, G., Nunziata, V., Malik, M. A., Poole, G. W. and Joplin, G. F., *Br.Med.J.,* 1976, **2,** 1473.

Papapoulas, S. H., Clemens, T. L., Fraher, L. J., Lewin, I. G., Sandler, I. M. and O'Riordan, J. L. H., *Lancet,* 1979, **i,** 627.

Serum Enzyme Disturbances

Fanburg, B. L., Schoenberger, M. D., Bachus, B. and Snider, G. L., *Am.Rev.Resp.Dis.,* 1976, **114,** 525.

Lieberman, J., *Am.J.Med.,* 1975, **59,** 365.

Selroos, O. and Klockars, M., *Scand.J.Resp.Dis.,* 1977, **58,** 110.

Intrathoracic Sarcoidosis

Hilar Adenopathy

Bein, M. E., Putman, C. E., McLoud, T. C. and Mink, J. H., *Am.J.Roentgenol.,* 1978, **131,** 409.

Smellie, H. and Hoyle, C., *Lancet,* 1957, **ii,** 66.

Winterbauer, R. H., Belio, N. and Moores, K. D., *Ann.Int.Med.,* 1973, **78,** 65.

Pleura

Wilen, S. B., Rabinowitz, J. G., Ulreich, S. and Lyons, H. A., *Am.J.Med.,* 1974, **57,** 200.

Gardiner, I. T. and Uff, J. S., *Thorax,* 1978, **33,** 124.

Chusid, E. L. and Siltzbach, L. E., 1974, **81,** 190.

Calcification

Scadding, J. G., *Tubercle,* 1961, **42,** 121.

Bronchial Stenoses

Citron, K. M. and Scadding, J. G., *Thorax,* 1957, **12,** 10.

Honey, M. and Jepson, E., *Br.Med.J.,* 1957, **2,** 1330.

Westcott, J. L. and Noehren, T. H., *Chest,* 1973, **63,** 893.

Chest Pain

Hendrick, D. J., Blackwood, R. A. and Black, J. M., *Br.J.Dis.Chest,* 1976, **70,** 206.

Myocardial Sarcoidosis

Ghosh, P., Fleming, H. A., Gresham, G. A. and Stovin, P. G., *Br.Heart J.*, 1972, **34**, 769.

Cor Pulmonale

Battesti, J. P., Georges, R., Basset, F. and Saumon, G., *Thorax*, 1978, **33**, 76.

Bone Sarcoidosis

Neville, E., Carstairs, L. S. and James, G. D., *Q.J.Med.*, 1977, **xlvi**, 215.

Nervous System

Matthews, W. B., *Br.Med.J.*, 1959, **1**, 267.

Matthews, W. B., *J.Neurol.Neurosurg.Psychiat.*, 1965, **28**, 23.

Douglas, A. C. and Maloney, A. F. J., *J.Neurol.Neurosurg.Psychiat.*, 1973, **36**, 1024.

Delany, P., *Ann.Int.Med.*, 1977, **87**, 336.

Skeletal Muscle

Douglas, A. C., Macleod, J. G. and Matthews, J. D., *J. Neurol. Neurosurg. Psychiat.*, 1973, **36**, 1034.

Joints

Gumpel, J. M., Johns, C. J. and Shulman, L. E., *Ann. Rheum.*, 1967, **26**, 184.

Parotid Gland

Greenberg, G., Anderson, R., Sharpstone, P. and James, G. D., *Br.Med.J.*, 1964, **2**, 861.

Upper Respiratory Tract

Neville, E., Mills, R. G. S., Jash, D. K., McKinnon, D. M., Carstairs, L. S. and James, G. D., *Thorax*, 1976, **31**, 660.

Oral

Bertram, U. and Hjörting-Hansen, E., *Scand.J.Dent.Res.*, 1970, **78**, 295.

Tarpley, T. M., Anderson, L., Lightbody, P. and Sheagren, J. N., *Oral. Surg.*, 1972, **33**, 755.

Hillerup, S., *Int.J.Oral.Surg.*, 1976, **5**, 95.

Kidney

Ford, M. J., Anderton, J. L. and McLean, N., *Postgrad.Med.J.*, 1978, **54**, 416.

Macserraigh, E. T., Doyle, C. T., Twomey, M. and O'Sullivan, D. J., *Postgrad.Med.J.*, 1978, **54,** 528.

Liver

Neville, E., Piyasena, K. H. G. and James, G. D., *Postgrad.Med.J.*, 1975, **51,** 361.

Rudzi, C., Ishak, K. G. and Zimmerman, H. J., *Am.J.Med.*, 1975, **59,** 373.

Eye

James, G. D., *Am.J.Med.*, 1959, **26,** 331.

Skin

Hancock, B. W., *Br.Med.J.*, 1972, **2,** 706.

Scadding, J. G., *Rapports du symposium européen de la sarcoidose,* Geneve, 1971.

Prognosis

Scadding, J. G., *Br.Med.J.*, 1961, **2,** 1165.

3. Diffuse Pulmonary Alveolar Fibrosis

With only a few exceptions, conditions giving rise to diffuse pulmonary alveolar fibrosis remain ill understood from the aetiological point of view. This has given rise to a great deal of confusion in the literature and numerous titles for the condition have been designed to try to embrace all of the variations. Regretfully, the inventors of these titles have not always used their terms precisely, thus perpetuating the confusion. Here diffuse pulmonary alveolar fibrosis means widespread fibrosis in that part of the lung beyond the terminal bronchioles which is concerned with gas exchange. Table 3 outlines the broad groups defined either aetiologically or histopathologically, and is included to serve only as a guide to conditions that may have to be considered in differential diagnosis. It will also be seen that several of the diseases mentioned have already been considered.

Cryptogenic Fibrosing Alveolitis

At present it is only possible to define cryptogenic fibrosing alveolitis histopathologically, although the diagnosis can be strongly suspected clinically and physiologically. In 1935, Hamman and Rich reported the presence of unusual pathological findings in four patients who all died of 'progressing suffocation'. They drew attention to the cardinal histological features of cellular thickening of the alveolar walls, together with fibrosis and the presence of large mononuclear cells within the alveolar spaces.

General Comments

The aetiology of cryptogenic fibrosing alveolitis remains unknown. Although the original cases of Hamman and Rich were all in younger people, it is known to occur in all age groups, but there is a greater preponderance in the sixth to seventh decade of life. The incidence of the disease would appear to be increasing. In part, this undoubtedly results from a greater clinical awareness. The cause is unknown, but there are similar conditions that result from exposure to various noxious agents. Cases of alveolar fibrosis have occurred during treatment with hexamethonium, busulpan,

Table 3. Diagnostic categories of pulmonary fibrosis.

Category	Examples and comment
Defined aetiologically	
Inhaled dusts	
Mineral	Asbestos and silica especially liable to cause alveolar fibrosis
Organic	Thermophilic actinomycetes— farmer's lung
	Avian antigens—bird fancier's lung
	Specific antigen—antibody reactions: hence the generic name 'extrinsic allergic alveolitis'
Ingested toxic substances	Paraquat, busulphan
Infections	
Bacterial	*M. tuberculosis*—chronic and healed Miliary tuberculosis
Fungal	Histoplasma, Coccidioides
Metazoal	Schistosoma, Filaria
? Viral	
Pneumocystis	
Defined histopathologically	
As part of a systemic disease with similar histology	
Sarcoidosis	
Histiocytosis X (eosinophilic granuloma)	
Mesodermal dysplasia (tumerous sclerosis)	
As a pulmonary disease	Most cases can be placed in a range
Fibrosing alveolitis	between 'desquamative' and 'mural' histological patterns. A few with unusual features can be appropriately designated. The pulmonary fibrosis associated with scleroderma, and that occurring in a few cases of rheumatoid arthritis, is a predominantly mural fibrosing alveolitis.

Reproduced with the kind permission of Professor J. G. Scadding.

bleomycin and methotrexate. There may be a genetic factor in some cases, since there is a higher incidence of the disease in certain families, twins and siblings. A recent report has shown an increased incidence of HLA-B12 in cyptogenic fibrosing alveolitis, but this was based on a small number of cases.

Clinical Manifestations and Disease Progress

The clinical hallmark is breathlessness. The presenting picture may be acute/subacute or chronic with reference to the rapidity of the progress. However, since the development of breathlessness is to some extent a subjective assessment and variable with age, it is often difficult to date the onset of the disease. In consequence, patients often relate the onset to irrelevant injuries or minor upper respiratory tract illness which may not have any bearing on the pathogenesis of the condition.

In acute/subacute cases, as described by Hamman and Rich (1944), the illness may be preceded by an acute infection with pyrexia and purulent sputum. The course of the disease is rapid and is measured in months. The patients rapidly become acutely breathless, sometimes complaining of chest tightness, but in all cases they eventually become tachypnoeic and cyanosed. Cough may be a troublesome feature. Such patients are often subject to episodes of acute worsening of their condition the cause for which is not apparent. They may improve within minutes or hours, but never return to normal.

In these patients the rapidity of the onset of the disease may lead to difficulty in diagnosis. Pneumonia and left ventricular failure may give rise to similar features, but appropriate treatment for these conditions will not lead to improvement here. As the disease progresses cor pulmonale supervenes and the patient becomes markedly cyanosed and oedematous.

Clubbing may develop in acute/subacute cases, but often the rapid progress of the illness does not allow this to become a marked feature. In all patients bilateral diffuse crackles are audible in the lung fields. These usually persist throughout the course of the illness. Occasionally bronchial breathing may be present, but may represent superadded infection. Patients usually die within six months.

In the chronic type of presentation early diagnosis can be difficult because not all the features may be present at the beginning. Again, difficulty in dating the onset is often experienced. Initially patients are breathless only on exertion, but eventually they are affected while at rest. Cough, in our experience, can be a considerable problem for the patient. Usually this is irritating and unproductive, and is precipitated by movement or change of atmosphere. It can lead to severe paroxysms which may be very tiring. Treatment of this problem can be very difficult. Cyanosis, again present only on exertion in the early stages, eventually supervenes in all cases. As the disease progresses, patients are more liable to secondary viral and bacterial infections, which lead to temporary worsening of symptoms together with purulent sputum production. Often such infections are a terminal event. Small haemoptyses may occur but are not usually serious or life threatening.

Finger clubbing occurs, the incidence varying between 30 and 70 per cent in the reported series. Hypertrophic osteoarthropathy has been described in association with the disease. Crackles are audible in both lungs, usually more marked towards the bases. In the early stages there may be marked asymmetry of these signs. Superadded infections will give rise to the appropriate clinical signs.

Investigations

Since the disease is defined histopathologically, lung biopsy remains the most important investigation. There are various techniques employed to obtain the specimens. Percutaneous methods using either drills or needles carry with them a significant complication rate, the main one being pneumothorax. In addition, the amount of tissue obtained is sometimes insufficient to reach a definitive diagnosis. Transbronchial biopsies with the flexible fibre bronchoscope have the same disadvantages in terms of specimen size, although the complication rate is much lower. More often than not, therefore, open lung biopsy has to be performed. This has additional advantages in that it permits a naked eye inspection and allows biopsies to be larger and, if necessary, to be taken from more than one place.

Haematological and biochemical tests have no specific diagnostic features in individual cases, although statistically it is possible to demonstrate differences from normal in a number of tests. Polycythaemia may occur, usually in those patients in whom cyanosis and oxygen desaturation are present. Eosinophilia sometimes occurs, although the differential diagnosis should be considered carefully if this is found. A raised ESR is not uncommonly encountered and this is probably related to an increase in the gamma globulins. This is usually due to a selective rise in IgA, IgM or IgG, although more than one may be elevated. Non-organ-specific antibodies are frequently present. Rheumatoid factor and antinuclear factor have been found present in up to 50 per cent of cases in some series. Antimitochondrial and antismooth muscle antibodies may also be present in the blood of these patients, although the incidence is lower than that of the antinuclear factor and rheumatoid factor. The frequent presence of these antibodies is in contrast to the low incidence in extrinsic allergic alveolitis.

Physiological abnormalities are usually demonstrable from the time the patient has symptoms. The vital capacity is reduced and the total lung capacity is low, but the residual volume is often well preserved. Due to the fibrosis in the lungs, they become less inflatable and stiff. This gives rise to a reduced compliance, because of the ensuing increase in elastic recoil and an abnormal negative transpulmonary pressure. For the same reasons the airways resistance is lowered due to the fibrosis holding open the small airways. This is reflected in a normal to increased ratio of forced expiratory volume in one minute to vital capacity.

The most consistently altered finding is a reduced diffusing capacity for oxygen and carbon monoxide. The transfer factor (measured during a single breath or in the steady state) is a measure of a number of different functions. It depends on the rate of gas transfer across the alveolar membrane (Dm), the blood volume of the pulmonary capillary bed (VC), and the ventilation perfusion ratio. Since all of these may be altered in cryptogenic fibrosing alveolitis to a greater or lesser extent, the transfer factor is a useful method of assessing the severity and progress of the disease. Finally, the control mechanisms of the lung tend to offset all of these defects by increasing the respiratory rate. Whilst this will maintain an adequate minute volume the physiological dead space is also increased, leading to an even greater defect in ventilation perfusion balance.

Recently broncho-alveolar lavage has been performed on a number of patients with cryptogenic fibrosing alveolitis. With this technique it is possible to obtain cells directly from the bronchial lining. The tests can be performed more than once on the same patient allowing changing patterns of cell counts to be studied. In the case of cryptogenic fibrosing alveolitis there appears to be an abnormally high number of neutrophils present in the lavage fluid and possibly of lymphocytes as well. Already, it has been suggested that such findings may be used to predict the patient's response to corticosteroids.

Radiology

There may be several different radiological appearances. Many attempts have been made to correlate radiological abnormalities with pathological findings; unfortunately these are not consistent enough to be useful diagnostically. In the acute/subacute type of disease or in desquamative interstitial pneumonitis of Liebow, extensive patchy shadowing, confluent in places and more extensive in the lower zones, was thought to correlate with the desquamative histological picture. In the chronic cases mottling occurs more frequently, and this was thought to relate to the mural histological picture. In both acute and chronic cases, however, too many exceptions occur. In the case of mottling, when it is very fine it may have a ground glass appearance. More often the mottling is more discrete with individual opacities measuring up to 2 mm in diameter.

As the disease progresses these opacities become coarser and rounded transradiances start to appear, which may vary in size from 5 to 10 mm in diameter. These are thought to represent bronchiolar dilatation. In all cases the shadowing tends to be more towards the bases. Serial radiographs often show a progressive shrinkage of lung size with a reduction in vertical height. This shrinkage may be asymmetrical, giving rise to unfolding of the aorta, kinking of the trachea, displacement of a fissure or shift of the mediastinum. The disposition of the shadows in the lower zones makes interpretation of heart size difficult due to lack of clarity of the heart border (Figure 17).

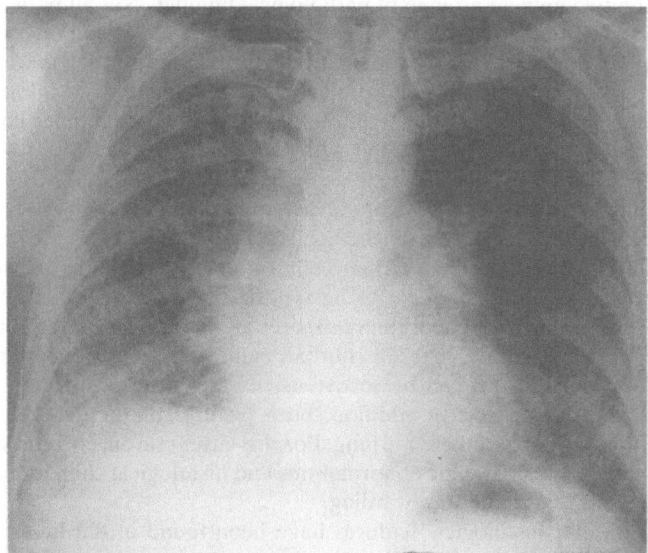

Figure 17. *Cryptogenic fibrosing alveolitis. Classical changes of diffuse micronodular shadowing more marked towards the bases with loss of clarity of the heart border and distortion of the trachea.*

Bronchograms show a diminution in the peripheral unfilled zone so that the bronchi filled with contrast material extend to the chest wall. There is bronchiolar and bronchial distortion.

Although very rare, cases have been seen with small rounded dense bodies mainly in the lower zones; these are due to small deposits of bone sometimes with marrow cavities. Finally, it must also be remembered that cases have been described where there is unequivocal lung biopsy evidence of the disease and the radiographs are normal.

Pathology and Immunology

Since this disease relies for definition on the histological findings, many pathological descriptions are available from reference. For convenience these have been reduced to two groups, representing the two ends of a range of pathological findings. Not all patients can be fitted into them perfectly. These groups have been referred to as the mural and desquamative types. In the former there is marked cellular thickening of the alveoli with lymphocyte infiltration together with collections of lymphoid tissue sometimes containing germinal follicles but without alveolar exudate (Plate 4). In the latter there is diffuse thickening of the alveolar walls with an infiltration of inflammatory cells, predominantly lymphocytic cells but with little established collagen. The alveolar spaces are filled with large mononuclear cells with clear eosinophilic cytoplasm which are thought to be type II pneumocytes (Plate 5). Between these two extremes mixtures are found more often than not, with more marked fibrosis and collagen deposition. Occasionally this can be so extensive as to render histological diagnosis difficult. In addition, both pictures may be found in different parts of the same lung. For this latter reason, correlation between radiographic abnormalities and histological changes has been difficult and unrewarding.

Similar histological features have been found in the lungs of patients suffering from rheumatoid arthritis, systemic sclerosis, Sjögren's syndrome and coeliac disease. In the case of rheumatoid arthritis patients with this lung complication, the arthritic component of the disease may not be troublesome and of only minor inconvenience. Careful questioning of patients with cryptogenic fibrosing alveolitis reveals that many admit to vague and variable arthralgic symptoms. In addition to these clinical observations, positive rheumatoid factor and antinuclear factor has been noted in some patients (see above) in whom there is no clinical evidence of these other diseases. Other diseases thought to have an abnor-

mal immunological basis have been reported to coexist with cryptogenic fibrosing alveolitis viz: Raynaud's disease, ulcerative col-
itis, thyroid disease, myelosclerosis, purpura, pernicious anaemia,
chronic active hepatitis, folic acid deficiency, myositis, adult
coeliac disease and renal tubular acidosis. All of these associations
logically suggest that altered immunological mechanisms may be
important in the development of cryptogenic fibrosing alveolitis.

It has been possible to demonstrate anticomplementary activity
in lung biopsy specimens, together with nonspecific antibody
activity. However, attempts at demonstrating definitive antilung
antibodies have been unimpressive. In vitro lymphocyte sensitiza-
tion to nuclear extracts has been demonstrated, but the interpretation of this still remains unclear.

In summary, there is some circumstantial clinical and labora-
tory evidence suggesting that abnormal immunological mechanisms play a part, if not in the aetiology then in the pathogenesis of
this condition.

Natural History

The early reports of cryptogenic fibrosing alveolitis suggested that
it was rapidly fatal. However, we now know that this is uncommon
and the usual course is one of steady decline over a number of
years. Occasionally the condition may arrest for a while, the
patient neither improving nor worsening. We have seen a small
number of cases of elderly people in whom histological diagnosis
has not been possible in view of their age and whose (presump-
tive) disease seems static. Such patients have very obvious radiographic and clinical abnormalities.

Treatment

Corticosteroids have been shown to be effective in certain
patients. Unfortunately clinical criteria cannot be laid down which
will predict which patients will respond. Care must also be taken in
assessing patients receiving corticosteroid drugs, because subjective improvement noted by the patient cannot always be corrobo-
rated by either functional or radiographic examination. Further, it

has been suggested that a better response can be expected in cases where little established fibrosis can be demonstrated histologically. Since great variation in the type of disease (i.e. mural or desquamative) and the amount of fibrosis can occur in the same patient, in practical terms it is not possible to predict the overall histological picture from biopsy material, or consequently, the response to treatment.

The immunosuppressive agents cyclophosphamide and azathioprine have also been used. In general, if these drugs are effective, it is in those patients who respond to corticosteroids. For this reason they may be helpful when used in combination with corticosteroids in smaller doses, thereby reducing the steroid side effects.

Penicillamine has also been tried in an effort to limit the amount of collagen tissue laid down. It is too early yet to say if this is effective and further studies are awaited.

Complications

The major complication of cryptogenic fibrosing alveolitis is respiratory failure. This is the commonest terminal event, and is often precipitated by superadded infection.

Cardiac failure may also occur as a terminal event; this was a marked feature of the acute cases noted in the original description. Bronchial carcinoma occurs more frequently in cryptogenic fibrosing alveolitis even allowing for the smoking habits of the patients. All cell types of bronchial cancer have been found.

Extrinsic Allergic Alveolitis

There are many agents which may give rise to extrinsic allergic alveolitis. However, the archetypal and first described example was that due to mouldy hay occurring in farm workers and often referred to as farmer's lung. Other synonyms such as thresher's lung, harvester's lung and hemp disease have also been coined. This condition, first described by Cadham (1924) in Canada and later was described more comprehensively by Campbell (1932)

and Fawcett (1936, 1938) in England following the handling
and close contact by workers with rain-soaked hay that had
been stored in badly ventilated conditions. It is now recognized as
a compensatable disease in the UK. Since then, many other antigens have been described which produce a similar disease (Table
4).

The illness varies widely in clinical acuteness and severity.
Classically, the patient presents with dyspnoea several hours after
being exposed to the offending antigen. This is usually associated
with marked constitutional symptoms. Fever, rigors, sweating,

Table 4. Nature and sources of organic dust antigens in extrinsic allergic alveolitis.

Disease	Dust exposure	Nature of antigen to which antibodies shown
Farmer's lung	Mouldy overheated hay	Thermophilic actinomycetes *Micropolyspora faeni Thermoactinomyces vulgaris*
Bird fancier's lung	Pigeon and budgerigar droppings	Avian serum protein antigens
Humidifier pneumonitis (Humidifier fever)	Contaminants of air conditioning systems	Thermophilic actinomycetes ? others
Maltworker's lung	Mouldy barley or malt	*Aspergillus fumigatus Aspergillus clavatus*
Bagassosis	Mouldy overheated sugarcane bagasse	Thermophilic actinomycetes
Sequoiosis	Mouldy redwood sawdust	*Aureobasidium (Pullularia) pullulans*
Maple bark pneumonitis	Maple bark	*Cryptostroma (Coniosporium) corticale*
Pituitary snufftaker's lung	Powder of porcine and bovine posterior pituitary extract	Serum proteins and pituitary antigens

muscle aches and pains and headache may be present collectively or in any combination. If attacks are repeated over a period of days or weeks, weight loss may become a striking feature. Sputum production may occur and even be bloodstained, but this is unusual. In the more chronic cases the constitutional symptoms are less marked. Wheezing, although not a common symptom, may occur particularly in those patients who continue to be exposed to the antigen for long periods of time.

Clinical signs consist of diffuse crackles throughout the lungs and in all the phases of respiration. Cyanosis may be present even at rest, particularly in the acute situation. Clubbing can occur but it is unusual and it is associated with the chronic stages of the disease.

Chest radiograph abnormalities may, and usually do, occur. In the acute cases fine micronodular shadowing is present sometimes giving rise to a ground grass appearance. This is usually confined to the middle and lower zones. Occasionally, larger patchy opacities may be present (see Figure 18). In chronic cases non-specific irregular patchy opacities or honeycombing may be seen.

Physiologically, these changes are associated with a fall in total lung capacity and a proportionate fall in FEV and VC. However, there is much greater and disproportionately larger fall in the gas transfer measurements, particularly in the acute illness.

Differential Diagnosis

Little can be confused with this condition if the patient presents with the classical symptoms following exposure to a known antigen. Unfortunately sometimes the symptoms may be inconsistently associated with exposure and under such circumstances careful history taking, with a full description of the patient's occupation and hobbies, may be necessary.

Pathology and Immunology

Pathologically, various changes may be found. The earliest and least often seen is that of pulmonary oedema. This is accompanied by interstitial lymphocytic infiltration. As the oedematous phase resolves, interstitial fibrosis appears. These changes are associated

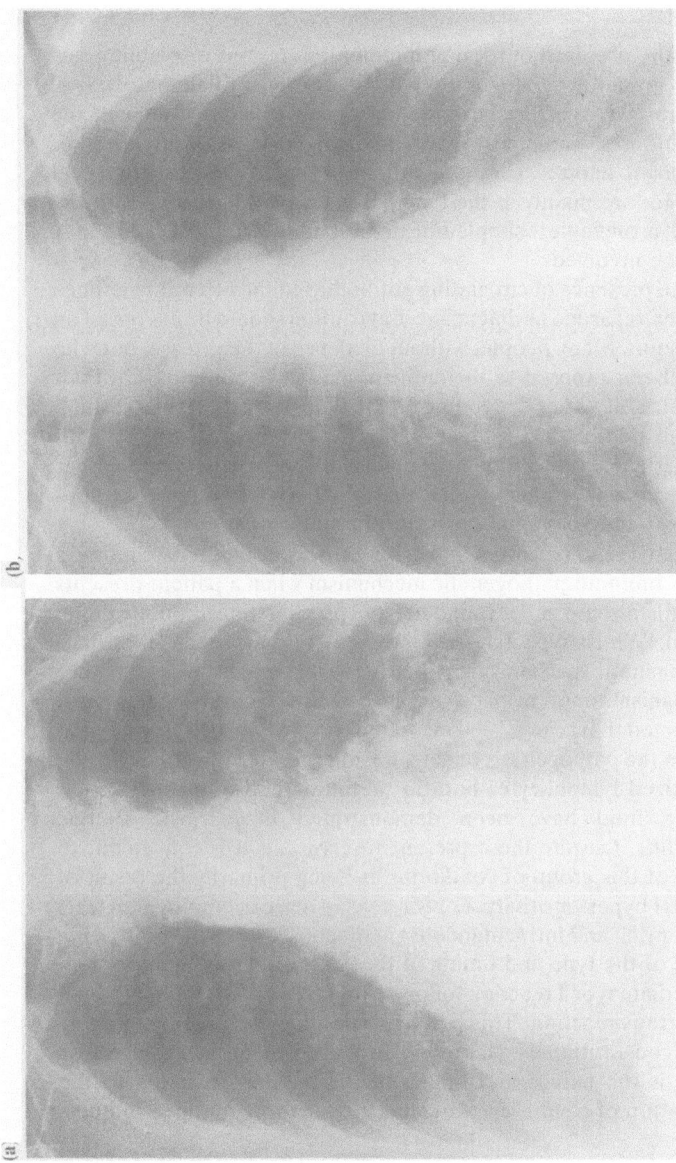

Figure 18. Extrinsic allergic alveolitis—budgerigar fancier's lung. (a) Diffuse patchy shadowing throughout the right lung, and to a lesser extent left lung. (b) Three months later, there is total clearing, no treatment other than removal of offending birds being necessary.

with the presence of focal granulomatous lesions resembling sarcoid granulomas, together with a chronic inflammatory cell infiltrate. Large foreign body-type giant cells are found in the granulomas, and these may contain pale translucent fibres of unknown nature. They are not birefringent. The pathological changes are mainly in the lung parenchyma, but the walls of the small bronchioles, subpleural tissue and interlobular septa may also be involved.

The presence of circulating antibodies to the offending antigen is often regarded as diagnostic, but caution should be exercised on this point. Many people, without evidence of the disease, but who have been exposed to the antigen, may have antibodies in their serum. This varies depending on the type of alveolitis in question. For example, the correlation between the presence of anti-budgerigar serum antibodies and disease in the case of budgerigar fancier's lung is much higher than the correlation between anti-farmer's lung hay antibodies and farmer's lung.

Even greater caution must be expressed before assuming a direct immuno-pathogenetic mechanism when a patient presents with the disease and is found to have precipitating antibody in the serum. Whilst type III Arthus reactivity may be an important pathogenetic mechanism giving rise to this form of disease, other mechanisms may also be involved. More recently it has been suggested that type IV cell mediated reactivity plays an important role in the pathogenesis of extrinsic allergic alveolitis. Specifically sensitized lymphocytes both in the blood and broncho-alveolar lavage fluid have been demonstrated in extrinsic allergic alveolitis. Despite these present reservations it is convenient to think of this group of conditions as being primarily the result of type III hypersensitivity. For this reason one can employ skin tests (both prick and intracutaneous) in diagnosis, a careful note being made of the type and timing of the reaction. Usually there is an immediate type I reaction followed four to six hours later by a type III Arthus reaction. This latter reaction may be accompanied by mild constitutional symptoms. Probably of greater diagnostic value is the nature and timing of the patient's reaction to the inhalation of a suitably extracted sample of the antigen in ques-

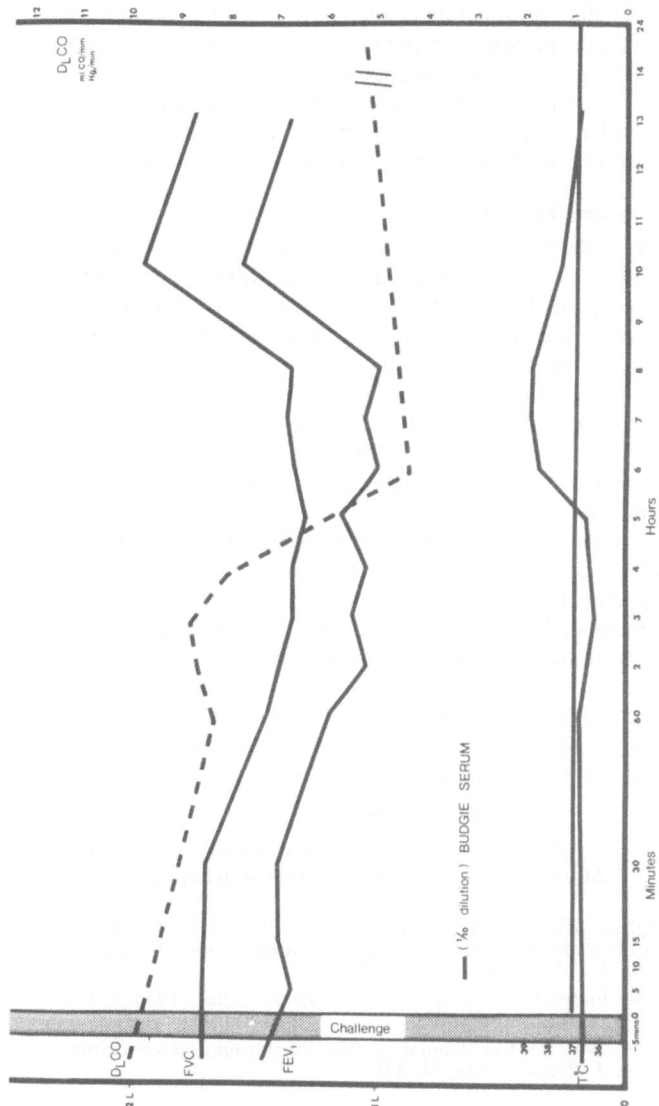

Figure 19. *Graphical record of patient following bronchial inhalation challenge using diluted budgerigar serum. There is a parallel fall in FEV_1 and FVC together with a fall in diffusing capacity (D_{LCO}), i.e. in a restrictive defect. This occurs concurrently with a rise of the patient's temperature starting four to five hours after challenge and lasting up to 12 hours.*

tion—bronchial provocation challenge tests. Great care must be exercised in the performance of these tests (Figure 19). The value of bronchial provocation challenge is not only in the isolation of the particular antigen but in the production of a mild form of the disease under investigation. In a limited way, therefore, a causal relationship between the antigen and disease is established.

Prevention and Treatment

Unchecked, these diseases can be fatal. However this is unusual for a number of reasons. Often the patient will be aware of the agent causing the disease and will therefore avoid it. If he has not already discontinued exposure to the offending agent, advice from his doctor will usually be accepted.

Two notable examples of exceptions to this situation should be mentioned. The authors have personal experience of the disease failing to remit and leading to death even after avoidance of the antigen. In the case of budgerigar fancier's lung, the very low concentration of antigen to which the patient is exposed usually does not give rise to symptoms until there is irreversible fibrosis, and avoidance of the antigen thereafter does not always give rise to improvement.

Treatment should consist of removal of the offending antigen. In this way, if the patient's condition improves, a casual relationship is established once again.

Occasionally, in severe acute involvement, corticosteroids may be administered to bring about a more rapid resolution of the symptoms and radiographic abnormalities.

Further Reading

Cadham, F. T., Asthma due to grain dusts, *J. Am. Med. Ass.*, 1924, **83**, 27.

Campbell, J. M., Acute symptoms following work with hay, *Br. Med. J.*, 1932, **2**, 143.

Eppler, G. T., McLoud, T. C., Gaensler, E. A., Mikus, J. P. and Carrington, C. B., Normal chest roentgenograms in chronic infiltrative lung disease, *N. Engl. J. Med.*, 1978, **298**, 17, 934.

Fawcett, R., Fungoid conditions of the lung, *Br. J. Radiol.*, 1935, **9**, 172, 354.

Fawcett, R., Vol. I. Occupational diseases of the lung in agricultural workers. *Br. J. Radiol.*, 1938, **11**, 378.

Hamman, L. and Rich, A. R., Acute diffuse interstitial fibrosis of the lungs, *Bull. Johns Hopkins Hosp.*, 1944, **74**, 177.

Liebow, A. A., Steer, A. and Billingsley, J. G., Desquamative interstitial pneumonia, *Am. J. Med.*, 1965, **39**, 369.

Pepys, J., Hypersensitivity disease of the lungs due to fungi and organic dusts. In *Monographs in Allergy 4*, P. Kallos, H. C. Goodman, M. Hasek, T. Inderbetzin and B. H. Waksman (Eds), Karger, Basle, 1969.

Scadding, J. G., Chronic diffuse interstitial fibrosis of the lungs, *Br. Med. J.*, 1960, **1**, 443.

Scadding, J. G., Diffuse pulmonary alveolar fibrosis, *Thorax*, 1974, **29**, 271.

Scadding, J. G. and Hinson, K. F. W., Diffuse fibrosing alveolitis (diffuse interstitial fibrosis of the lungs). Correlation of history at biopsy with prognosis, *Thorax*, 1967, **22**, 291.

Stack, B. H. R., The clinical manifestations and diagnosis of fibrosing alveolitis, *Tubercle*, 1971, **1**, 15.

Turner-Warwick, M., Cryptogenic fibrosing alveolitis, *Br. J. Hosp. Med.*, 1972, **7**, 697.

Turner-Warwick, M., Haslam, P. L., Lukoszek, A., Townsend, P., Allan, F., Du Bois, R. M., Turton, C. W. G. and Collins, J. V., Cell, enzymes and interstitial lung disease, *J. R. Coll. Phys.*, 1981, **15**, 5.

4. Honeycomb Lung

Honeycomb lung is a radiological term indicating the presence of multiple cysts, usually throughout both lungs. These cysts vary in size from 5 to 20 mm in diameter, and they represent the end point of a number of different disease processes. The diseases which may give rise to this radiological appearance are: diffuse alveolar fibrosis (described on page 65), histiocytosis X, tuberous sclerosis and Von Recklinghausen's disease (neurofibromatosis).

Histiocytosis X

In 1893 Hand described a three-year-old boy with exophthalmos, polyuria, hepatosplenomegaly, lymphadenopathy and an area of bone destruction of the skull. Reports of a similar disease followed from Schuller (1915) and Christian (1920) and later this became known as the Hand–Schuller–Christian syndrome (HSC syndrome).

Shortly afterwards, Letterer (1924) and Siwe (1933) described a rapidly fatal disease of children characterized by fever, hepatosplenomegaly, lymphadenopathy and bone lesions. In 1940 Lichtenstein and Jaffe published a report of an apparently self-limiting disease characterized by the presence of isolated bone lesions.

The histological feature which is common to each of these conditions is infiltration of the tissue by histiocytes. This led Lichtenstein (1953) to suggest that all three conditions were part of a single entity, which he named histiocytosis X. Although of similar pathology, the clinical manifestations of each syndrome are varied. This has caused some authors to question whether they are not separate diseases, rather than variants of the same disease. Until the aetiology of this condition is known, this question will remain unsolved.

Pathogenesis

The microscopic appearance of a lesion from any site is of an infiltrate of histiocytes, which may be markedly lipidized (foam cells), accompanied by varying numbers of mature eosinophils. In solitary bone lesions large numbers of eosinophils may be present. Engelbreth-Holm et al. (1944) suggested that the pathological process went through four phases: an initial proliferative histiocytic stage (with no foam cells), a granulomatous stage, a xanthomatous stage with large numbers of foam cells and a healing fibrotic stage.

Clinical Features

Letterer–Siwe syndrome

Characteristically, this syndrome occurs in the first year of life with the rapid development of fever, weight loss and anaemia. Diffuse pulmonary infiltration, hepatosplenomegaly and lymphadenopathy may occur. Skin lesions, which may be papular, petechial or erythematous, are common. The outcome of the disease is usually fatal, death resulting from marrow failure, respiratory failure or septicaemia.

Hand–Schuller–Christian syndrome

This syndrome usually occurs in childhood, approximately 70 per cent of cases presenting under the age of 15 years. It is twice as common in males as in females. The classical triad of exophthalmos, diabetes insipidus and bone lesions is relatively uncommon. Children present with either a palpable mass over a bone lesion, polyuria or skin rashes.

Bone lesions are found in almost all patients with this disease. The lesions may occur at any site, but are most commonly seen in the skull, scapula, ribs, pelvis and the long bones of the arms and legs. They may be asymptomatic, but often give rise to pain. Lesions of the mastoid and petrous temporal bones are frequently associated with otitis media. Exophthalmos may result from a tumour mass originating either within the orbital cavity or in its walls. Proptosis may be unilateral initially, but usually becomes bilateral.

Pulmonary involvement occurs in about one quarter of cases and may be confined to the lungs alone. Various terms have been used for this latter disease, including eosinophilic granuloma of the lung, primary pulmonary histiocytosis X and primary pulmonary eosinophilic granuloma. Pulmonary symptoms tend to be minor, patients presenting either as a result of a routine chest radiograph or more commonly with symptoms of a nonproductive cough and exertional dyspnoea. Rarely acute symptoms of fever, anorexia, pleurisy and night sweats are present. Complications of pulmonary involvement include spontaneous pneumothoraces, progressive pulmonary fibrosis and cor pulmonale.

Eosinophilic Granuloma of Bone

The bone lesions are similar to those of HSC syndrome. In the original description (Lichtenstein and Jaffe 1940) this is a benign disease of children and young adults, with no associated symptoms or signs and with a tendency to spontaneous resolution in the majority of patients. Single or multiple bone lesions are seen. When the lesions are multiple, other features of HSC syndrome are more likely to be present.

Radiological Features (Figure 20)

The appearance of the bone lesions is of sharply demarcated osteolytic lesions which are round or oval in shape. When healing takes place, the lesions may undergo sclerosis. The pulmonary abnormalities are typically bilateral diffuse nodular shadows. The densities vary in size from 2.0 to 4.0 mm in diameter, but occasionally larger nodules are present which may cavitate. These appearances may progress to diffuse interstitial fibrosis and honeycomb lung. Hilar lymphadenopathy rarely occurs.

Pulmonary Function Tests

In only a few publications have the abnormalities of lung function in histiocytosis X been reported. These have shown evidence of a mild restrictive defect with little impairment of diffusing capacity.

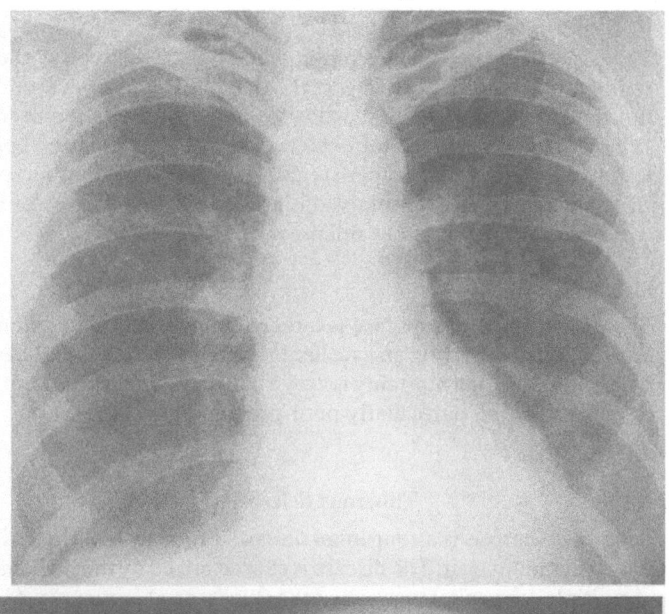

(a)

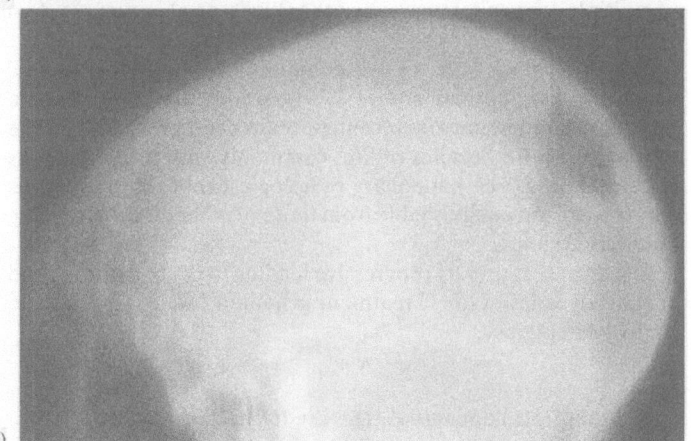

(b)

Figure 20. *Histiocytosis X. Radiographs of a 42-year-old female presenting with breathlessness. (a) Honeycomb shadowing is present throughout both lung fields. (b) Tomography of her skull reveals a well circumscribed osteolytic lesion in the right occipitoparietal region.*

Diagnosis and Treatment

The association of bone lesions combined with the typical chest radiograph changes may suggest the diagnosis of histiocytosis X, but to establish a definite diagnosis a tissue biopsy is required.

Treatment depends on the extent of the disease. Localized bone lesions respond well to either surgical curettage or radiotherapy. In disseminated disease remissions are initiated in most cases by corticosteroid therapy, but relapses are frequent.

Prognosis

The prognosis of this disease is largely determined by its extent, solitary lesions carrying an excellent prognosis. When the disease is disseminated, the mortality is very high; and skin involvement is associated with a particularly poor prognosis.

Tuberous Sclerosis

Tuberous sclerosis is a congenital disease, probably inherited as a single dominant trait. The disease is characterized by the presence of multiple congenital tumours of the skin, central nervous system and viscera.

The presenting features are commonly epileptic fits, mental deficiency and fibroadenomas of sebaceous glands (adenoma sebaceum). Pulmonary involvement may occur, presenting in the second and third decades of life, commonly with a spontaneous pneumothorax. The pulmonary radiological changes in tuberous sclerosis are indistinguishable from those of other diseases causing honeycomb lung.

The disease is usually progressive leading to death in the second or third decades of life. Treatment is limited to the symptomatic control of epilepsy.

Von Recklinghausen's Disease (Neurofibromatosis)

Von Recklinghausen's disease is inherited as an autosomal dominant. It is characterized by multiple tumours of craniospinal nerves and pigmentation of the skin. Honeycomb lung occasionally complicates this disease.

Further Reading

Histiocytosis X

Lieberman, P. H., Jones, C. R., Dargeon, H. W. K. and Begg, C. F., *Medicine*, 1969, **48**, 375.

Engelbreth-Holm J., Teilum G. and Cmristensen E., *Acta Medica Scandinavica*, 1944, **292**, 118.

Lichtenstein L. and Jaffe H. L., *American Journal of Pathology*, 1940, **16**, 595.

5. Interstitial Pulmonary Changes in Some Systemic Diseases

In this chapter, the clinical features of four disorders will be discussed:

1. Amyloidosis.
2. Systemic lupus erythematosus.
3. Rheumatoid disease.
4. Progressive systemic sclerosis.

Amyloidosis

Amyloidosis is not a single entity, but a group of protein deposition disorders. The first descriptions were of amyloidosis associated with chronic sepsis and chronic tuberculosis, especially of lung and bone; later, a primary form and similar types, associated with myelomatosis and other plasma cell dyscrasias, were identified. Several heredofamilial and tumour-associated forms have since been described.

Protein Deposition

Until the advent of electron microscopy, the deposition of protein appeared homogeneous and had characteristic tinctorial properties with certain dyes, e.g. Congo red. It is now known that the major constituents of amyloid deposition are protein fibrils (the amyloid fibrils).

In cases of primary amyloidosis and that associated with myelomatosis, the major protein in the deposition has been shown to be a homogeneous light polypeptide chain (Lc) or its amino terminal variable (VL) fragment of a light chain from an immunoglobulin molecule.

In amyloidosis secondary to chronic sepsis, tuberculosis,

rheumatoid disease and familial Mediterranean fever, the major protein fibril (AA) in the deposition is of non-immunoglobulin origin. The cellular origin of these AA proteins is not known. In these cases, the major sites of protein deposition are the liver, spleen, kidney and adrenals. Liver cell dysfunction is uncommon, but proteinuria, the nephrotic syndrome, renal vein thrombosis and uraemia may be the main clinical features.

In primary amyloidosis, the protein deposition may result in dysfunction of many organs, and thus the clinical features of primary amyloidosis may simulate a number of other diseases. In the gastrointestinal tract, the tongue may be relatively immobile, and be so enlarged that it is permanently protruded because the oral cavity is too small to accommodate it. The surface of the tongue may be nodular or furrowed. The oesophagus, stomach and intestines are commonly sites of deposition; pyloric narrowing may occur and the intestines may be converted into thickened rigid tubes. In the heart, deposition is common and may be the cause of death. The heart is usually enlarged and comparatively rigid; clinically there is congestive heart failure with diminished myocardial movement and on the ECG tracings low voltage ventricular complexes are the main features.

Renal, ureteric and bladder involvement may result in proteinuria, renal failure, frequency of micturition and dysuria.

The peripheral nervous system is frequently involved in primary amyloidosis; muscle weakness, paraesthesiae, numbness, intractable postural hypotension and impotence have all been well documented.

Skin deposition, which is sometimes extensive, may result in the presence of nodules or plaques either opaque or translucent. An associated purpura may give rise to palpable purpura, especially around the eyes. Amyloid deposition may result in generalized lymph gland enlargement, replacement of haemopoietic tissue in bone marrow, painful swollen joints, contractures of fingers and para-articular nodules, especially around the shoulders and elbows. In the region of the wrist joint, deposition may cause a carpal tunnel syndrome.

In the respiratory tract, amyloidosis may be a localized

deposition in the tract itself, or may be part of a widespread deposition in many tissues.

Where amyloidosis is localized in the respiratory tract, the deposition may be present as a localized tumour or tumours. The commonest site is the larynx, although deposition also occurs in the nasal sinuses, trachea and the bronchi. When the bronchial lumen is occluded by an amyloid tumour, the clinical and radiological features may resemble bronchial carcinoma or bronchial carcinoid. In addition, amyloid deposition may be widespread in the tracheal and bronchial mucosa, with or without amyloidosis in other organs.

Multiple nodular pulmonary amyloidosis may also be a localized lung disorder or be part of a widespread disease (Figure 21).

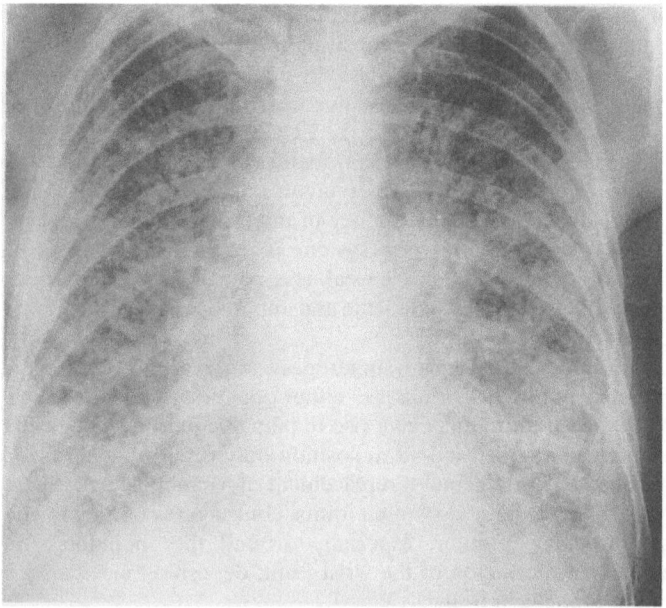

Figure 21. *Primary nodular pulmonary amyloidosis.*

The pulmonary nodules may be numerous, small and discrete, or the deposits may coalesce, rendering a lobe or lobes solid. The deposits may even extend to the mediastinal connective tissue and mediastinal lymph glands. In the cases where the nodules are confined to the lung, the prognosis may be good. Diffuse alveolar septal amyloidosis is usually associated with amyloid deposition in many organs. Shortness of breath, a defective gas transfer and the presence of bilateral diffuse reticulonodular shadows on the PA chest radiograph are the main features of this pulmonary form of the disease. The prognosis in these cases is poor (macroglossia, heart, skin and peripheral nervous system involvement may also be found).

In a small minority of cases of myelomatosis and closely allied plasma cell dyscrasias, amyloid deposition occurs in a distribution similar to that of primary generalized amyloidosis (Figure 22). In the cases of myelomatosis, there is nearly always Bence Jones

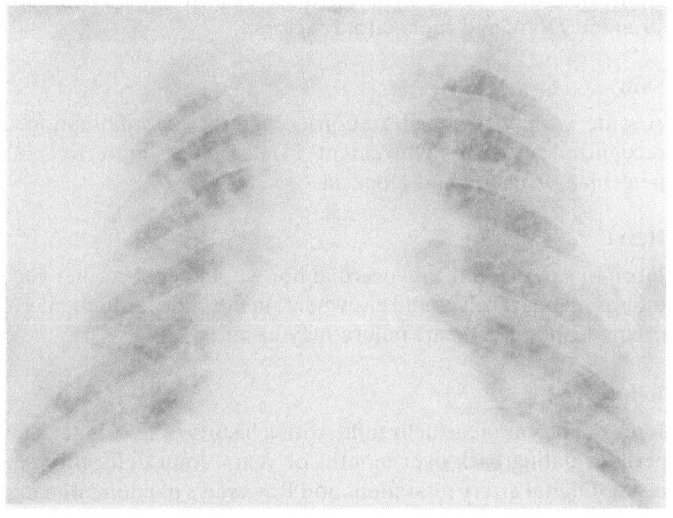

Figure 22. *Amyloidosis of the lungs in a case of myelomatosis.*

(light chain) proteinuria present and seldom a great increase in the serum globulin levels. Thus, in myelomatosis, congestive heart failure, arthropathy, peripheral neuritis, macroglossia, bowel symptoms and diffuse lung changes may result, singly or in combination, as a result of an associated amyloid deposition.

Systemic Lupus Erythematosus

Systemic lupus erythematosus (SLE) usually affects many systems. Although its aetiology is unclear, there is evidence that it is an autoimmune disorder, i.e. there is an inappropriate production of an immune response against self antigens. The damage caused by this response may result in fibrinoid deposition. This change particularly involves the intima of arterioles. Secondary inflammatory changes with formation of collagen occur.

The abnormalities in the immune system are reflected in a number of changes which can be demonstrated in the serum, e.g. antinuclear antibodies, including those against single and double stranded DNA and rheumatoid factors.

Skin

A wide variety of manifestations, singly or in combination, is recognized in skin involvement in SLE, e.g. butterfly rash, petechiae, urticaria and alopecia.

Heart

Fibrinous pericarditis, myocardial fibrosis and endocardial vegetations on heart valves and elsewhere on the endocardium may all occur. Congestive heart failure may ensue.

Joints

Joint symptoms are usually mild, with a history of transient aches, perhaps dating back over months or years. Joint deformity may result. Digital artery infarctions and Raynaud's phenomenon may occur.

Muscle aches and muscle tenderness are common.

Kidney

Kidney involvement may be evident by the presence of proteinuria, oedema due to protein loss in urine and renal failure. Renal involvement is important as a prognostic indicator; it is associated with a poor outlook.

Nervous System

Peripheral neuropathy, epilepsy, hemiplegia and mental disturbances may all result from arteritis involving cerebral vessels.

Gastrointestinal Tract

Recurrent abdominal pain, sometimes very severe and sometimes even without tenderness, may be a dominating feature of gastrointestinal tract involvement; diarrhoea and gastrointestinal bleeding may occur.

Respiratory Tract

Pleurisy is common in respiratory tract involvement, and pain may be the presenting symptom, which may be very severe. Persistent bilateral pleural effusions may occur, which may be large and occasionally be associated with a pneumothorax. Sometimes pleural pain, with or without a pleural rub, may persist for many months. In such cases, a pleurectomy may result in great symptomatic relief.

In the lung itself, atelectasis, with or without bronchial obstruction by mucus, is common. The cause of this is unclear—an abnormality of surfactant activity has been suggested.

Undue shortwindedness may occur without radiographic abnormalities of the lungs, apart from 'raised' diaphragms (noted on the PA chest radiograph). Again, the cause of this symptom is unclear, but the presence of interstitial pulmonary changes, not sufficiently large to result in changes on the PA chest radiograph, is likely. Such changes include alveolar septal oedema, inflammation and hyaline membrane development. It is now known that marked functional derangement of the lung, associated with definite histological changes of interstitial lung disease of various origins, may occur in the absence of radiographic abnormalities in

the lung. In SLE radiographic evidence of interstitial lung disease
is uncommon.

Rheumatoid Disease

Formerly, this condition was called rheumatoid arthritis, because
a major feature of this illness is often a bilateral, inflammatory
and, eventually, a destructive condition of joints, especially the
peripheral ones. It is now recognized as a generalized disease
which may involve several systems.

The disease affects females more often than males, with a peak
incidence in the fifth decade of life. The aetiology remains
obscure. Although certain infective agents, both bacterial and
viral, have been held responsible, none has been proven.

An outstanding feature of rheumatoid disease is the overactiv-
ity of the immune system as shown by first, the presence of
lymphocytes and plasma cells in the synovial membrane; second,
the presence of rheumatoid factors in the serum (these factors are
immunoglobulins directed against determinants on other
immunoglobulins); third, the demonstration of intracellular
immune complexes in synovial fluid removed from affected joints.

In rheumatoid disease, apart from the polyarthritis, there may
be:

1. Evidence of arteritis involving small vessels in nail folds or
larger arteries to fingers or bowel.

2. Constitutional symptoms and signs, including fever, weight
loss, sweats, malaise, anaemia and occasionally, in long-standing
cases, secondary amyloidosis with the protein deposition in the
liver, spleen, kidney and adrenals.

3. Various forms of peripheral neuropathy occur, including
mononeuritis multiplex and symmetrical peripheral neuropathy.

4. Scleritis.

5. Subcutaneous nodules, usually on extensor aspect of the fore-
arms or tendo achilles. These nodules are usually bilateral,
multiple, non-tender and mobile.

Respiratory Tract

It is now recognized that several manifestations of rheumatoid disease may occur: pleural effusion, fibrosing alveolitis and lung nodules.

Pleural Effusion

Pleural effusion is usually unilateral and sterile on culture. It may precede or accompany the better known polyarthropathy.

Fibrosing Alveolitis

The features of fibrosing alveolitis (interstitial lung disease) are very similar to those of cryptogenic fibrosing alveolitis: usually, a history of increasing shortwindedness, where patients often complain of their being unable to fill their chests fully with air. Dry, short cough is a common symptom and later in the illness tachypnoea, may be noted. On examination, apart from the distress of the dyspnoea and the tachypnoea, there are, on auscultation, fine crackles heard; these crackles are usually more evident at the bases of the lungs and are more often bilateral, but are sometimes unilateral.

Finger and toe clubbing develop in most cases; hypertrophic osteoarthropathy is a rare complication. The functional abnormalities reveal, as expected, restriction and a marked defect in oxygen transfer.

Chest radiographic abnormalities, usually bilateral and more marked at the lung bases, comprise reticulation, nodulation and a honeycomb appearance (Figure 23). Occasionally, the radiographic appearances are more marked on one side than the other. There is no close correlation between the degree of radiographic abnormality on the one hand and the extent and profusion of the crackles on the other.

Lung Nodules

Lung nodules are uncommon but when they do occur they are often sited under the pleura. They may be single or multiple, rounded in the outline and may measure up to 5 cm in diameter.

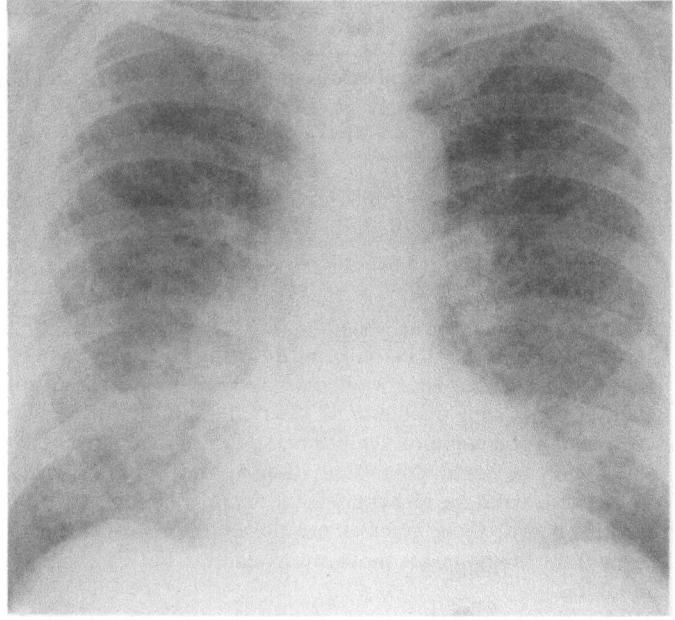

Figure 23. *Interstitial lung disease in a case of rheumatoid disease.*

The lesions may cavitate. The chest radiographic appearances may simulate a peripheral lung cancer.

In coalminers who suffer from pneumoconiosis and rheumatoid disease (Caplan's syndrome, see page 19), widespread, fibrotic nodules may develop in both lungs and these lesions may precede the other features of rheumatoid disease. The lesions may calcify, cavitate or, following cavitation, the cavity itself may disappear radiologically.

In addition to pleural effusion, lung nodules and fibrosing alveolitis, there is probably an increased incidence of chronic bronchitis in rheumatoid diseases. This is sometimes severe, with widespread bronchiectatic changes as sequelae.

Progressive Systemic Sclerosis

Progressive systemic sclerosis (PSS) is a disease of unknown aetiology, sometimes called scleroderma because of the conspicuous involvement of the skin in most, but not all, cases. The disease may also involve the heart, kidney, lung and gastrointestinal tract, especially the oesophagus. Females are more frequently affected than males. The usual age of onset is 35 to 50 years, but it may present in childhood.

In the skin, the fingers become stiff with reduction in volume of the pulp, the result being a firm, tapered fingertip—sclerodactyly is the term used for these changes.

Deposits of calcium salts in the fingertips, especially in the pulp, may occur. These deposits may ulcerate through the skin and be extruded. Similar deposits may occur in the region of the elbows. Facial changes in PSS are characteristic—a tight mouth, thin lips and furrows in the skin running from the mouth, both in upper and lower lips. Telangiectasia may be a prominent feature. The skin changes may involve arms and trunk. Polyarthritis of the hands may occur in early cases.

Raynaud's phenomenon commonly precedes, sometimes by years, the other features of PSS.

Gastrointestinal Tract

Involvement of the oesophagus in PSS is common and may be demonstrated at an early stage of the disease. Symptoms comprise dysphagia, heartburn (due to incompetence of the cardia), recurrent cough and episodes of bronchitis or pneumonia due to spillover of oesophageal contents into the trachea and bronchi.

Barium swallow examination may show the presence of a dilated, atonic oesophagus, even before the development of dysphagia, heartburn, etc.

Other parts of the gastrointestinal tract may be involved and give rise to duodenal ileus, malabsorption and diarrhoea.

Heart

Patchy replacement of the myocardium by fibrosis may be associated with congestive heart failure and dysrhythmias, including bundle branch block. Cardiac enlargement may occur and may be secondary to hypertension, a sequela of renal damage by the disease. A pericarditis may also occur.

Kidneys

Damage to the kidneys with renal failure and hypertension is a common cause of death in PSS. The amount of proteinuria bears no constant relationship to the severity of the kidney damage.

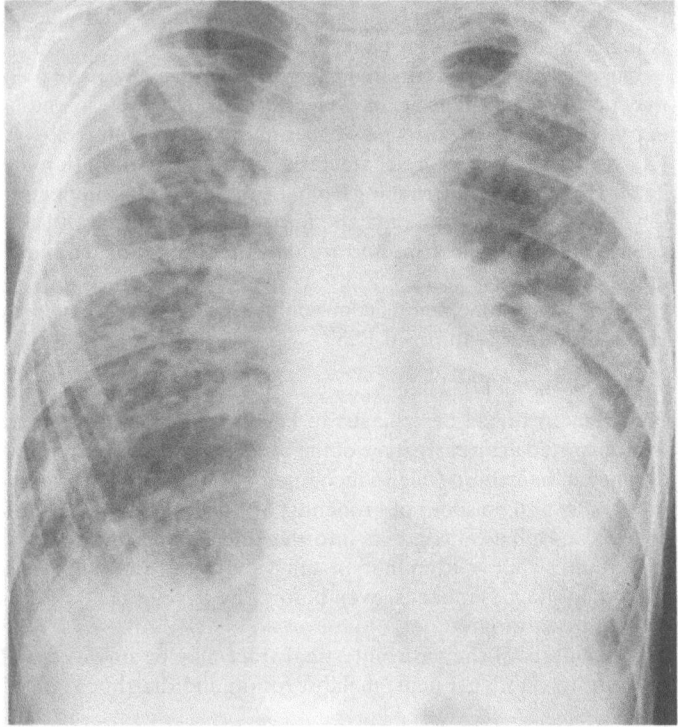

Figure 24. *Severe pulmonary changes in a 14-year-old boy with progressive systemic sclerosis. The face, hands, heart, oesophagus and kidneys were all involved.*

Lungs

The lungs are involved in about one third of cases of PSS. Post-mortem examination shows the presence of intra-alveolar and interstitial fibrosis. These changes may be accompanied by the development of a honeycomb appearance due to the presence of cysts (Figure 24). Peribronchial and pleural fibrosis, the latter often marked, are common.

Patients, like those with SLE, may complain of shortness of breath and may have a functional abnormality (restrictive pattern and diffusion defect) without any radiographic abnormalities. However, when radiographic changes are present, they are usually more conspicuous at the bases and consist of nodulation and/or linear shadowing, and honeycomb appearances may be evident. In addition to shortness of breath, other features are cough, bilateral basal crackles, and recurrent pulmonary infections due to spillover from the oesphagus, when this is involved by the disease. Adenocarcinoma of the lung may develop in PSS.

Further Reading

Crofton, J. and Douglas, A., *Respiratory Diseases*, 2nd Edition, Blackwells Scientific Publications, Oxford, 1975, Ch. 34.

Gordon, W., Amyloid deposits in the bronchi, *Br.Med.J.*, 1955, **I**, 825.

Hobbs, J. R., An ABC of amyloid, *Proc.R.Soc.Med.*, 1973, **66**, 705.

Lee, S-C. and Johnson, H. A., Multiple nodular pulmonary amyloidosis, *Thorax*, 1975, **30**, 178.

Mason, M. and Currey, H. L. E., *An Introduction to Clinical Rheumatology*, 2nd Edition, Pitman Medical, 1975, Ch. 2, 7 and 8.

Poh, S. C., Tzia, T. S. and Seah, H. C. Primary diffuse alveolar septal amyloidosis, *Thorax*, 1975, **30**, 186.

Scheinberg, M. A. and Cathcart, E. C., New concepts in the pathogenesis of primary and secondary amyloid disease, *Clin. Exp. Immunol.* 1978, **33**, 185.

Spencer, H., *Pathology of the Lung*, 3rd Edition. Pergamon Press, Oxford, 1977, Ch. 19.

Symmers, W. St. C., Primary amyloidosis: A review, *J. Clin. Path.*, 1956, **9**, 187.

Symmers, W. St. C., Five cases of primary generalised amyloidosis, *J. Clin. Path.*, 1956, **9**, 212.

6. Pulmonary Fibrosis Associated with Pulmonary Eosinophilia

Any discussion of pulmonary fibrosis associated with eosinophilia poses a number of problems. Although pulmonary fibrosis occurs in association with pulmonary eosinophilia, it is not known if the former results from the latter, or if both are an expression of an as yet unknown underlying pathogenic mechanism. In addition; the classification of pulmonary eosinophilia is to some extent a retrospective one made when sufficient time has elapsed to exclude the development of known disease with which it be associated.

Eosinophilia can be associated with a number of respiratory diseases or systemic diseases which involves the respiratory tract as part of that disease process, causing widespread fibrosis within the lung tissue. A peripheral eosinophilia cannot always be demonstrated even when pathological examination of the tissues in question shows extensive eosinophilic infiltration. Because of this it is possible that the condition of pulmonary eosinophilia occurs more frequently than has been reported. As a result of these difficulties, an arbitrary definition of pulmonary eosinophilia has to be used; i.e. chest radiographic abnormalities occurring in association with a peripheral blood eosinophilia, providing other causes for the shadowing or eosinophilia are not present. Other causes might be, for example, infection occurring in an asthmatic patient who has a concurrent peripheral eosinophilia, hydatid disease or Hodgkin's disease. A number of other names have been used to refer to this group of conditions. Loeffler's syndrome is occasionally used to refer to this broad group when, in fact, even the author was only describing one small specific entity of transient pulmonary shadowing with an associated peripheral eosinophilia. In the American literature the term 'PIE' is sometimes used to mean *pulmonary infiltrations* with a blood eosinophilia. A number of these conditions will not be discussed here and are mentioned for the sake of completion. Asthma is sometimes associated with pulmonary eosinophilia and forms the basis of a broad classification shown in Table 5.

Bronchial asthma can, and often does, have an associated peripheral blood eosinophilia. However, radiographic shadowing is unusual, although it may occur. Under such circumstances a syndrome of pulmonary eosinophilia with asthma is recognized. Within this category broad distinctions can be made such that it is possible to anticipate the pathology, and thereby act as a guide to the natural history of the disease and its treatment. The syndrome may occur in asthmatic patients who are atopic extrinsic or non-atopic intrinsic. The former group accounts for approximately 80 per cent of the syndrome and is usually caused by hypersensitivity to the common mould *Aspergillus fumigatus*. This is called allergic bronchopulmonary aspergillosis. The hypersensitivity gives rise to episodes of repeated radiographic abnormalities which may be associated with an increase in asthmatic symptoms together with constitutional upset. Fever, muscle aches and pains and purulent sputum production may occur. The sputum may also be blood-stained and often contains 'plugs'. These are hard pieces of a gelatinous substance which, when examined microscopically, are found to contain the septate branching hyphae of the mould.

The distribution of the radiographic shadowing is variable not only between patients but also in the same patient at different times. Many different types of shadows have been described. When not confined to a whole lung, lobe or segment the shadowing is often perihilar with shaggy borders having no obvious anatomical relationships. This type of shadowing has been shown not only to give rise to persistent fibrotic change, but also to the development of a particular type of bronchiectasis, wherein the dilatation occurs midway along the bronchi giving rise to the so-called proximal bronchiectasis. The cardinal feature of this is that on bronchographic examination the draining bronchi and bronchioles beyond the bronchiectatic area are normal. It is thought that the damaged areas of the bronchi are where the antigen–antibody reactions have occurred. Great variations in the degree of residual fibrosis may occur; some patients seem to suffer

Table 5. Classification of pulmonary eosinophilia.

Atopic status	Aetiological agent	Treatment	Comment
Pulmonary eosinophilia with asthma			
Atopic	*A. fumigatus*	Corticosteroids, either intermittently or continuously	Range of host variation from those of low atopic to high atopic status. Precipitating antibody present
Atopic	Unknown	May require corticosteroids	Variable atopic status
Non-atopic	Unknown	Corticosteroids	So called cryptogenic pulmonary eosinophilia — some may progress to polyarteritis nodosa
Pulmonary eosinophilia without asthma			
Non-atopic	1. Helminths, e.g. Ascaris, Toxocara, Filaria	Appropriate antihelminthic agent	Complement-fixing or immunofluorescent antibody test often positive
	2. Drugs – nitrofurantoin, antituberculous drugs, gold antibiotics	Withdrawal of offending agent. Occasionally corticosteroids	—
	3. Unknown	Corticosteroids	Cryptogenic pulmonary eosinophilia — some may progress to polyarteritis nodosa

only one or two episodes which leave only minor asymptomatic scarring, while others may have almost persistent 'active' shadowing which gives rise to progressive fibrosis and ultimately may lead to respiratory failure. For the most, however, there is a middle course. They are subject to exacerbations of the disease which only cause minor damage and lead to fibrosis only after many years (Figure 25).

Diagnosis of this condition rests upon the demonstration of the following:

1. Radiographic shadowing.

2. Positive skin prick tests to Aspergillus extracts.

3. A peripheral eosinophilia.

4. Usually some evidence of variable airways obstruction.

5. The presence of Aspergillus antibodies (precipitins) in the blood.

6. Sputum 'plugs' microscopically showing hyphae.

The problem of asthma and pulmonary eosinophilia in patients in whom no sensitivity to Aspergillus can be demonstrated gives rise to great difficulties in diagnosis. Often referred to as cryptogenic pulmonary eosinophilia, the diagnosis may well have to be kept under review for many years because a small proportion (approximately 10 per cent) of such patients develop evidence of polyarteritis nodosa. However, at presentation certain clinical and radiographic features may help. In such patients the peripheral eosinophilia is often very high; it may amount to 80 per cent of the total white cell count. The patients are often intrinsic asthmatics and their total IgE concentration is normal (in contrast to the group due to Aspergillus sensitivity, when the total IgE during an attack may be markedly elevated). Radiographically the shadowing is often peripheral, diffuse and hazy. The response to treatment with corticosteroids is quite dramatic even when only relatively low doses are used (15 to 30 mg prednisolone daily). Patients should always be carefully observed.

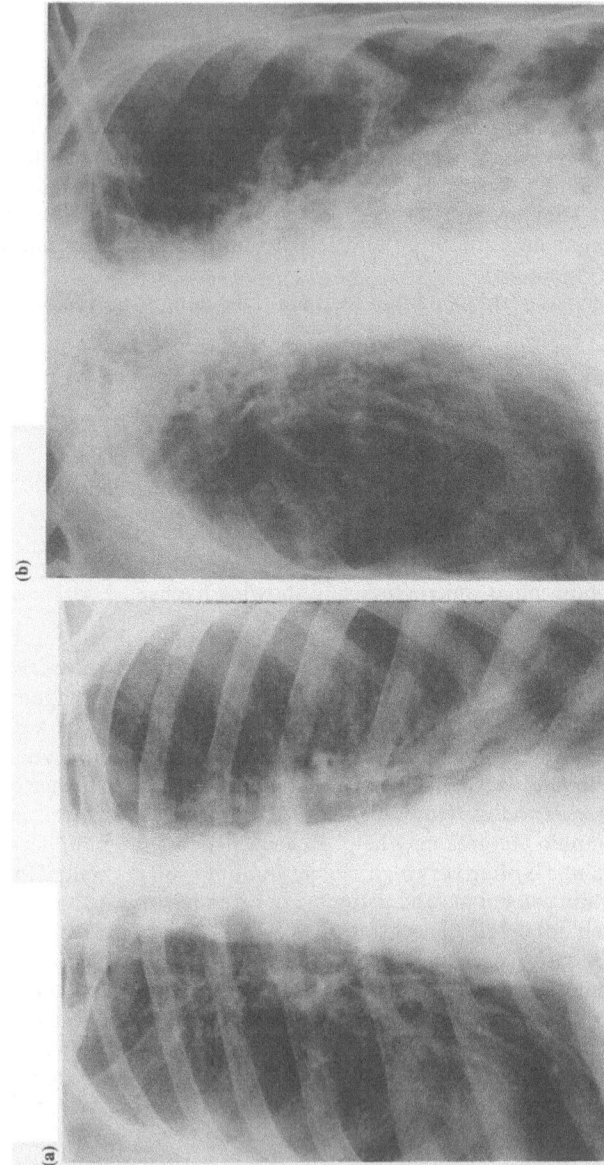

Figure 25. Allergic bronchopulmonary aspergillosis. (a) Only minimal shadowing in the right upper zone. (b) 23 years later, extensive fibrosis in both upper zones together with shadowing in the left lower zone.

Polyarteritis Nodosa

This may occur in patients with a previous history of airways obstruction, but it also occurs in the absence of such a history. Polyarteritis nodosa is an uncommon disease and often fatal. The lung is said to be involved in 30 to 40 per cent of cases. Great diagnostic difficulty can be encountered in trying to delineate between such conditions as cryptogenic pulmonary eosinophilia, polyarteritis nodosa, Wegener's granulomatosis, etc. Indeed, it is to be argued that separating such conditions into strict compartments is unrealistic because they may simply represent examples within a range of conditions. If one thinks of them in this way, it encompasses the great overlap of clinical presentation and pathology that one meets. Nevertheless, a broad separation has some merit in that it allows for better prognostic and treatment guidelines to be established. At all times the clinician should be prepared for great variation.

The aetiology is still not known. Due to the similarity between the florid presentations and serum sickness some authors feel that the pathological and clinical features result from immune complex deposition. In particular, when renal involvement occurs complement activation and depletion has been demonstrated. However, no consistent non-organ-specific or organ-specific antibodies have been found. Australia antigen has been reported with increased frequency in the disease, but surprisingly not when the lung seems to be involved. Drugs have been incriminated as a possible cause, particularly the sulpha groups, but the evidence for this is scanty, and only applies to a small number of cases.

When the lung is involved the incidence of eosinophilia is much higher than in those cases when it is not.

Pathology

The naked eye findings fall into two main groups. First, there may be necrotic and caseous-like areas resembling tuberculosis. These may be of any size, often appear nodular, involve any amount of a lobe or whole lung, and may even cavitate. They may be associated with haemorrhage into the alveoli. The disease process may also involve the large bronchi and trachea. Second, infarcts are commonly found; these may be of any size but have no distinguishing features. Occasionally, evidence of bronchiectasis may be found.

Microscopically, areas of eosinophilic infiltration may be seen, but they are not usually associated with the nodular lesions. These areas show tuberculosis-like lesions consisting of necrosis surrounded by giant cells, lymphocytes, plasma cells and neutrophils. The pulmonary vessels show proliferation of the intima and infiltration by neutrophils and eosinophils. In addition, fibrinoid changes are also found within the arteries and capillaries. Involvement of the small vessels seems to be a feature of polyarteritis when it affects the lungs. In other cases where the lungs are not involved larger vessels are usually affected.

Clinical Features

Polyarteritis nodosa may sometimes be preceded by a history of asthma or chronic bronchitis. When it occurs in association with asthma there seems to be a greater delay before other systems are involved, but in either situation the initial symptoms are those of an acute respiratory tract infection which fails to improve. Under such circumstances no objective evidence of an infecting agent is found and the patient usually fails to respond to antibiotics. Other patients tend to present with a picture of acute bronchitis with cough, wheezes and crackles. There is usually a high blood eosinophilia, especially in those patients with asthma where it may comprise up to 80 per cent of the total white cell count. The respiratory symptoms are usually associated with more constitutional symptoms such as weight loss, lethargy and weakness. As the disease progresses haemoptysis and pleuritic chest pain tend to occur. This may be the result of infarction or the breaking down of the consolidated areas which may produce a lung abscess. This latter development is often associated with secondary bacterial infections with such organisms as Proteus and Pseudomonas. Occasionally these may be the presenting symptoms. Effusions may also occur. Death may ensue as a result of any of these events.

General manifestations, such as weight loss, anorexia and lassitude, are often quite marked. Any system may be involved in the disease process and this often gives rise to complex clinical pictures. Renal involvement is certainly the most serious complication because this often heralds a rapid decline in the patient's condition and is particularly unresponsive to treatment. The patient may present with a clinical picture not unlike acute glomerulonephritis with proteinuria, microscopic haematuria, hypertension, etc., and occasionally a nephrotic syndrome may occur. Gastrointestinal manifestations include bloody diarrhoea, infarction or perforation of some part of the gastrointestinal tract and malabsorption symptoms may occur. Neurological involvement can give rise to cranial nerve palsies, mononeuritis multiplex, polyneuritis or polymyositis, as well as cerebral symptoms resulting from involvement of the cerebral arteries. Rheumatological manifestations akin to rheumatic fever or rheumatoid arthritis can occur. Heart involvement is common—myocardial infarction, coronary insufficiency, cardiac failure and hypertension have all been described. Indeed, it is possible to find ECG abnormalities even without cardiovascular symptoms. Skin manifestations may be a presenting symptom and consist of small arteritic lesions like splinter haemorrhages, sometimes larger, giving rise to gangrene or purpura.

Radiology

The chest radiograph usually shows patchy opacities resembling pneumonic consolidation. The opacities do not necessarily conform to the natural anatomical boundaries and they may be transient, other shadows reappearing either in the same or different parts of the lung. Nodular shadows of all sizes from miliary to large rounded shadows, several centimetres in diameter, may occur and occasionally cavitate or form abscesses. Effusions may also occur.

Investigations

Diagnosis depends on biopsy evidence of the disease and muscle biopsy is usually the most appropriate. Although muscle groups which are not giving rise to symptoms may show evidence of the disease, most clinicians advise biopsy of those that have either clinical or electromyographic evidence of involvement.

In patients with lung involvement eosinophilia is said to occur in approximately 50 per cent. A leucocytosis is also commonly found. The gammaglobulins are usually raised, and so is the ESR. The antinuclear factor is only occasionally positive.

Natural History

This disease is usually fatal; however the time course may vary considerably. Lung involvement carries no worse a prognosis than when polyarteritis nodosa presents in other organs. Renal involvement is always a bad sign. Three months is the average survival time when multisystem involvement occurs.

Treatment

The mainstay of treatment is corticosteroids and the initial dose should be prednisone 40 to 60 mg daily, to bring the disease under control. Thereafter, the dose is reduced to control the disease activity. There is some evidence to suggest that swift resolution of the pulmonary opacities improves the outlook. Cytotoxics, such as methotrexate and cyclophosphamide, have been tried but no clear-cut advantage is apparent at the present.

Wegener's Granulomatosis

Regarded by many people as a variant of polyarteritis, this condition was first described by Wegener in 1936. The characteristic features are the presence of granulomas in the nasopharynx or antra, together with lesions in the respiratory tract, a generalized arteritis and a focal form of glomerulonephritis. A more localized form of the disease has been described where there are pulmonary lesions similar to those seen in the generalized form but no other components of the disease are present. However, since the pulmonary lesions can antedate the rest of the disease, it is difficult to know if this distinction represents a genuine difference. In the cases described as localized Wegener's disease the prognosis would appear to be a little better.

Clinically, patients with generalized disease have one or more of the following: persistent purulent rhinorrhoea, nasal obstruction, antral pains, epistaxis and proptosis. In some patients, pulmonary symptoms present first and consist of chronic cough, haemoptysis and chest pains together with breathlessness. Renal symptoms, comprising haematuria with or without pain, usually occur late in the disease. The urine is heavily loaded with protein and casts. Renal failure eventually supervenes and is the commonest cause of death.

Radiology

Features similar to those seen in polyarteritis nodosa are found. Waxing and waning shadows with or without cavitation are the commonest lesions (Figure 26).

Pathology

The involvement of the upper respiratory tract is the main differentiating feature. The lesions in the nose may lead to palatal or orbital perforation with destruction of the facial tissue near the root of the nose (midline granuloma). Meningitis as a consequence of this has been described. In the localized form pseudotumours of the orbit have been noted. The respiratory tract may be involved over its entire extent. Ulceration of the trachea and bronchi is common. In the lung, many creamy yellowish necrotic lesions are found. They vary in size and can resemble tuberculosis. The disease extends to involve any amount of the lung tissue and can reach the pleural surface which may be adherent to the chest wall. Haemorrhagic pleural effusions may be found. Microscopically, areas of infarction and granulomatous change are found. There is central necrosis surrounded by numerous giant cells of the Langhans type, together with acute and chronic inflammatory cell infiltration (Plate 6). Eosinophils may be present. In the infarcted areas at the edges of the lesions severe fibrosis is often found. In the nasopharynx spreading granulomas composed of plasma cells, lymphocytes and polymorph leucocytes may be found eroding the tissues. The renal lesion shows a picture of acute glomerulonephritis.

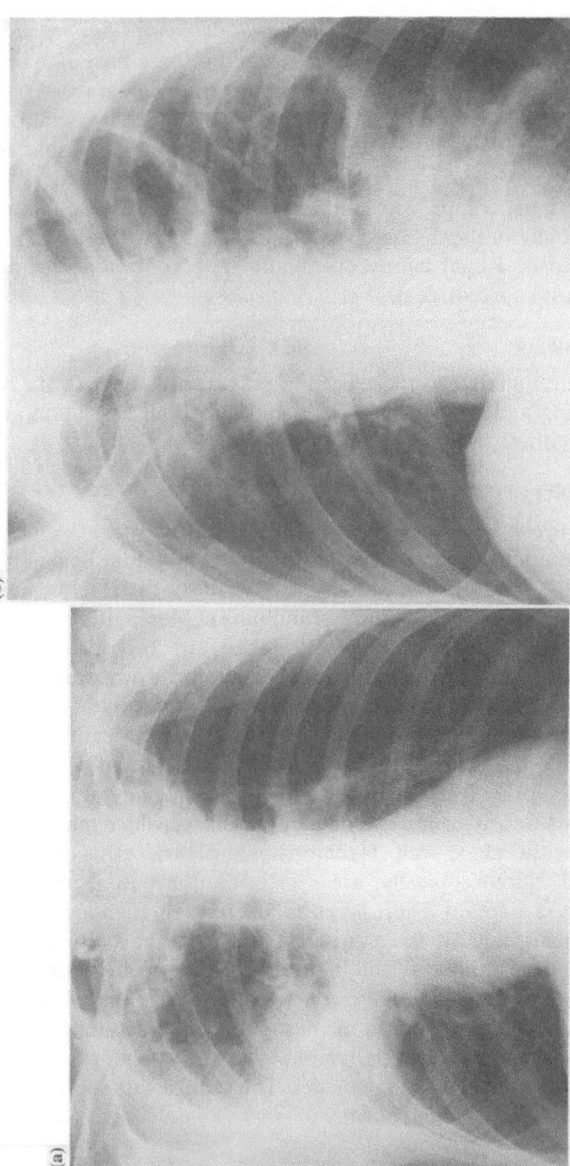

Figure 26. Wegener's granulomatosis. (a) An area of consolidation in the right midzone and a thick walled cavity in the right upper zone. (b) Two years later, two thin walled cavities have developed in the left lung.

Natural History

In the localized form of the disease spontaneous resolution has been described. In the generalized disease the time course depends very much on how quickly renal disease supervenes. Between one and two years without treatment is the usual survival time.

Diagnosis

Biopsy of affected organs remains the only method of diagnosis. Often nasal biopsies are sufficient.

Treatment

To date, corticosteroids administered in a similar way to that described for polyarteritis have been the mainstay. However cytotoxics, particularly cyclophosphamide and methotrexate, seem to be showing promise and early studies suggest a good first time remission rate when pulmonary lesions are the main problem. Although no definite direct evidence of immune complex activity has been demonstrated, some patients with pulmonary and renal lesions have been treated by cytotoxic therapy and plasmapheresis with good effect. However, insufficient cases have been described to be certain about the future role of plasmapheresis in treatment.

Tropical Pulmonary Eosinophilia

Left untreated this condition may give rise to fibrosis, although this is rare nowadays. The largest reported series of cases emanates from the Indian subcontinent, although cases have been described from Sri Lanka, Burma, Malaysia, tropical Africa, South America and the Southern Pacific. The condition is usually due to infection with the filarial parasite, although the pulmonary manifestations may be partly due to an allergic reaction to the parasite.

Clinically the disease usually starts with a dry irritating cough followed by wheezing. Fever is present in one third of cases and occasionally chest pain and haemoptysis occur. Physical signs are usually unhelpful consisting mainly of wheeze and inconsistent crackles. Chest radiographs usually show ill defined bilateral mottling sometimes coalescing to produce the picture of consolidation. Line shadows, pleural effusion and cavitation may also occur.

An absolute blood eosinophilia is always present and is usually in excess of 2000/mm^2. Total IgE levels may also be very elevated. A filarial complement fixation test is invariably positive. It is usual to perform stool examinations since many helminths can produce similar symptoms.

Treatment consists of the appropriate antihelminthic, usually diethylcarbamazine.

Further Reading

Carrington, C. B. and Liebow, A. A. Limited forms of angeitis and granulomatosis of Wegener's type, *Am. J. Med.*, 1966, **41**, 497.

Crofton, J. W., Livingstone, J. L., Olswald, N. C. and Roberts, A. T. M. Pulmonary eosinophilia, *Thorax,* 1952, **7**, 1.

Hinson, K. F. W., Moon, A. J. and Plummer, N. S. Bronchopulmonary aspergillosis. A review and a report of eight new cases, *Thorax,* 1952, **7**, 317.

Liebow, A. A. and Carrington, C. B. The eosinophilic pneumonias, *Medicine,* 1969, **48**, 451.

Rose, G. A. and Spencer, H. Polyarteritis nodosa, *Quart. J. Med. N.S.,* 1957, **26**, 43.

Scadding, J. G. Eosinophilic infiltrations of the lungs in asthmatics, *Proc. Roy. Soc. Med.,* 1971, **64**, 381.

Index